Something
to
Say

Wandering
Back to
Saskatchewan

CHARLOTTE EVELYN SLOAN

This novel is set in the province of Saskatchewan, Canada, with reference to fictitious prairie towns. The era covered is the 1930s - 1950s. The names and characters are fictional, and their involvement in the events and circumstances of this time period is a figment of the author's imagination.

This book is third in the series: Wandering Back to Saskatchewan.

ISBN 978-1-7778663-2-7 (Hardcover)
ISBN 978-1-7778663-0-3 (Paperback)
ISBN 978-1-7778663-1-0 (EPUB)
ISBN 987-1-7778663-3-4 (Kindle)

Editing & Proofreading Services, Lantern Hill Communications

Published by Marmie's Corner

First Edition: August 2021

Dedicated to my son, Kevin

Who did not give up.

CONTENTS

SOMETHING TO SAY

Fall sunshine bathes the farmyard in an ethereal glow of bright yellow, gold, and red. Peace and beauty mingle together as a feathery breeze rustles the leaves. Suddenly, the calm is shattered by a terrifying gunshot blast, the scream of a little girl, a loud clatter on wide, wooden floor planks, and the sobbing of a man.

Long legs with overalls flapping, gaining ground across the dried grass. Someone urgently yanks open the heavy barn door.

Far inside, at the back by the mangers, dim light reveals that the man who sobs is not a man, he is a bewildered teenager, a dark shock of long hair covers his face. The boy's eyes are closed, gulping air as he cries.

The girl, all arms and legs, huddles in the straw and clutches his shirt. She is in shock, eyes wide but unseeing. The man in overalls is down, reaching in the straw for both. He is the best choice, the very best choice if anyone were choosing who should come.

No one speaks. The rifle crack is now far away. Silence, except for the crying. The redhead pushes away the hands and she stands, unsteady and trembling.

"I said, Don't - don't die!"

"You said right, little girl. You said right."

The sun shines in through the cracks of the west wall. Dust motes shift in the shaft of light. Time passes. There is no urgency to move. A hand is bleeding - it is no matter. The girl stands like a statue, staring at the two who lie in the straw.

Three times she repeats: "I said, Don't - don't die!"

Each and every time she says it, the older man reassures her, "You said right. You said right!"

WHERE'S MY DAD?

Maggie Andersen had a lot to say when she started Grade 1. She had already turned six when she joined Hal and Dorie in the buggy, bound for the one-room Aroma School each weekday morning.

Laura, a girl in Grade 2, was snoopy and extra curious about the new redhead in Grade 1. She was not shy about asking questions. "How far do you live from school? Is Hal your brother? What's your Mom like? Do you have a Dad?"

Maggie promptly responded to all the inquiries but she was stumped for an answer regarding her Dad. Laura pressed further. "What happened to him? Ask your Mom, and then come back and tell us."

During the first week of school, the Grades 1s and 2s were let out fifteen minutes early before the noon hour, probably to give the teacher a bit of a reprieve. As they were still getting accustomed to the long school day, the extra playtime was welcome. The kids found lots to do while on the school grounds with no adult supervision. Some of them preferred to play games. A couple of the boys couldn't get enough of playing tag, running at full speed till their faces were flushed and sweaty.

Hoping to find a response for her interrogators, Maggie initiated an interesting conversation at the supper table. She looked at her mother and her siblings and asked innocently, "Where's my Dad?"

Her mother, Thea, gave her the look straight from Hades. Dorie, five years older than Maggie, was much more confident and braved the lion without fear.

"Oh come on, Maw, why won't you answer her? We don't remember him much, but we did have a Dad."

Hal grinned. He looked up from his corn and potatoes and said, "Maybe not, I think we just hatched from an egg like your chickens, Maw!" He was trying to be funny which Dorie didn't appreciate. She gave them all a knowing look and said, "Listen, every henhouse has a rooster."

Maggie was puzzled. The next day at school, the other students persisted. "So, where *is* your Dad? Did you find out what happened to him?"

Maggie answered as well as she knew how, and what she said seemed to satisfy the other children. "I think he got et up by a rooster."

MAGGIE'S HERO

Fred Fiske had finished Grade 8 a few years before. The year he quit, on the last day of June, he was happy to walk out of the schoolyard for the last time. He was taller than his father, big enough and old enough to take on his share of the farm work, and to plan for his future. He was building up a cow herd and dreamed of owning a farm soon. Fred was known as kind and easy-going, but there was an unspoken understanding that Fred was a guy you didn't push.

There are bullies the wide world over. What is it in some people that they feel entitled to be cruel? There were two classic bullies at the Aroma School and they clubbed together to torment the little kids and anyone else they took a notion to insult. Oliver Meyer was the meanest and Sam Holmes was almost his equal. They started throwing their weight around the day school started in the fall. They were not there for learning, and anyone could see they were up to no good. The inexperienced young teacher had a wide-eyed, scared look as she called the class to order each day.

Before the first week was over, Oliver had most of the little kids calling Hal's little sister "Maggie Rooster". Hal was no match for the bullies and so he ignored it, pretending he didn't hear their taunting. He well knew they were making fun of his mother's chicken farm as much as they were of his defenseless little sister, who once told the other kids at school that her Dad was killed by a rooster. When word came to Fred Fiske about what was going on over at the school, he lost no time driving the short distance to the school and confronting Oliver and Sam.

"Maggie, come here."

Maggie trotted over to Fred and the bullies, all smiles, knowing she would come to no harm with her neighbor protecting her. Fred stared them down. His look was level and threatening.

"This girl's name is Maggie Andersen. Don't you dare make fun of her or call her anything except her name. Don't even dream of it, or you'll answer to me."

The boys looked at each other with sheepish grins. They were probably more embarrassed than anything but before they knew what was happening, Fred's big hands grabbed each one by the front of the shirt. Those watching heard the sound of ripping cloth. Without a second thought, Fred knocked the boys' heads together. When he released them, they fell on the steps, dazed and blinking.

Fred swung Maggie up onto his shoulders and asked, "How do things look from up there, Maggie Andersen?"

She patted the top of his head. "Things look good, Fred. They look really good." From then on, Fred was her hero, and so was his brother, Bobby. The entire Fiske family was her saving grace.

FISKES AND ANDERSENS

The two families were destined to be more than friends, and more than neighbors. Life events would weld them together, creating a unique bond. The houses were situated across the road from one another, with a well-worn path from one door to the other. The same sun shone down on both farm yards each day and the same moon cast its light on them at night, but there the similarities ended.

Stanley and Bessie Fiske's farmyard was well-kept and orderly, featuring a good-sized barn, and a white frame house with a green door and matching shutters. A small porch provided room for boots and included a wooden washstand with an enamel washbasin for cleaning up after outside work. Coats, coveralls, and an apron hung on a row of convenient hooks on the inner wall, and a sheer curtain drawn to one side of the window revealed cheery red geraniums. They grew in a row of peanut butter cans on the sill.

Bessie Fiske eagerly opened her door to friends and strangers, and her trademark hospitality was well known for miles. "Well, come on in, and sit a spell!" was her usual greeting. Stanley and Bessie were well-matched. They had come to the prairies with their pioneer families and were proud of the farm they had built together. They had a reputation of hard work and generosity. Bessie liked to tell the story of how her father, John Stevens and his brother Alf, managed in a wild snowstorm, to find the pins buried in the ground, proving which homestead was theirs.

Bessie's thick, greying hair framed her girlish face and was kept in place with a hairnet. When she smiled, her face lit up like sunshine. Her eyes were bright and blue. Each day, she wore a two-pocket apron and an attached chain of safety pins. She laughed her way through her stories, as one of her finest gifts was her ability to see the lighter side of things. It was an essential trait to combat the harsh lifestyle of farming in those difficult years of the dry and thirsty Dirty Thirties, and the war years of rations and heartache.

Stanley was a farmer through and through - plaid shirt, denim overalls, and heavy boots. He was bald on top with a fringe of dark hair that Bessie kept trimmed with a good set of clippers, ordered from the catalogue. She regularly tamed his bushy eyebrows with her sewing scissors. She also took care of his gold-rimmed glasses that were usually in need of cleaning. When Stanley came in from outside, Bessie often held out her hand for the glasses and gave them a dip in the washbasin. A beat-up brown felt hat saved his bald head from sunburn, and his ready smile was the feature that made him approachable to all. The man possessed a fierce love for his wife and his boys. He had a tender, understanding heart, and it took a lot to get him worked up. Stubborn and loyal to the core, he was not a man you would want to cross on important issues.

Bessie and Stanley were overjoyed when they became parents. Fred was their firstborn, and six years later, along came Bobby. The boys were strong and solidly built, with round faces and straight, black hair. Fred was outgoing and friendly. Bobby was tentative and timid. Big brother was protective of little brother. The four of them played crokinole on winter nights, popped corn on the cook stove, and in an evening when the work was done, Bessie read aloud by lamplight. Sometimes she read a continuing story from the weekly paper, but her listeners preferred a few pages from one of her favorite books. *Helen's Babies* was a well-known comical story about a bachelor uncle who took care of his two young nephews. The book was enjoyed by the whole family and Bessie read it with gusto. They were a secure and happy family, working hard to combat the challenges of prairie hardships.

Across the road, life was not so sweet. A pleasant, treed lane led into the Andersen establishment, which gave the impression of a welcome and flourishing yard. But the minute the house came into view, the desolation and forlorn appearance of the old two-story house revealed a different picture altogether. Weathered shingles covered the exterior walls. It was a ramshackle dwelling, with a distinctly neglected air about it. The door had once been painted white, and an open porch leaned to the east. Three backless, cast-off wooden chairs were lined up, no doubt providing a cooler place to sit in summer when the house was hot.

The main outbuilding was a large henhouse, with a wire-covered chicken run that could provide shelter for a huge population of poultry. Thea Andersen sold eggs to the local stores and young fryers to the creamery. She hired a man to seed and harvest a crop on her quarter section of land. She sold most of the grain, but kept some for chicken feed. A couple of sheds were located side by side near the well. One was for the cow and the other was for the hired man who bunked there seasonally, spring to fall. In winter there was no need for hired help. The only chores were to milk the cow and keep the chickens going.

The place was not inviting in any way. There was no tea kettle whistling on the stove to offer a quick cup of tea to visitors. Thea ruled the roost, spent more time with her chickens than with her children, and her mouth naturally turned down on the sides.

Dorie and Hal were one year apart and Maggie, the youngest, lagged behind her brother by four years. Dorie coped at school by coming across as "high and mighty". She did well at academics, as did Hal. Little Maggie was another story. She did whatever she could get away with. The connection between the Andersen family members was thin, and you might say each of them lived alone, together, in that house.

Dorie was tall and slim, and overall was rather satisfied with her looks. She smiled to bring out the dimples in her cheeks, even if her smile was fake.

Hal was also quite taken with his looks and spent time in front of his dresser mirror, practicing his grin and slicking his straight, brown hair in whatever direction he thought looked most impressive. He was a fun-loving boy, always gunning for something new, and forever trying to make people laugh. He had a slight build and was a daredevil. Hal liked climbing high, whether up trees or on buildings, and he yelled when he wanted to, for no reason in particular. Since his mother hired a man to do the farm work, Hal looked for fun, rather than ways to help out. He was not very interested in work. Dorie constantly reminded her brother that he was a lazy son-of-a-gun. She called him that to his face, but Hal wasn't bothered by what people said to him.

Like most kids of that age, six year old Maggie was missing her two front teeth. Her eyes were a watery blue. Freckles from the whole summer were plastered layer on layer, across her face, which was topped by an unruly mop of red hair.

All her life, she had been scared of the dark and begged to spend the night in her sister's bed. Night after night, Dorie refused and ordered her back to her own bedroom. "Close your eyes and go to sleep. That's not so hard!"

Maggie protested, "But it's worse when I shut my eyes. That's when I see the specks of dark."

"You what?" There was no use trying to explain. Maggie waited until her sister was asleep and then noiselessly rolled up in a blanket on the floor. In the morning, the older sister had no mercy when she once again spied the rumpled blanket with red hair sticking out of it, right beside her bed. She dragged the quilt, girl and all, out of her room and closed the door.

One summer day, Maggie found a mouse nest while snooping in the hired man's bunk house. She knew she was in luck when she pushed back the soft, shredded mattress stuffing and viewed several tiny, pink bodies. She decided to keep them for pets and found a small pail to put the whole nest in. She carried them around for the afternoon and even poured water on them to cool them down. Finally, she left them on the buggy seat and by the time she thought of them again, they had disappeared! Her mother had just left the chicken pen, and Maggie ran to meet her.

"Do you know where my pets went?"

Thea looked puzzled.

Maggie anxiously added, "You know, my little friends. They were in a pail!"

Thea looked disgusted. "You mean those baby mice? They're no pets! I just fed them to the hens."

Maggie was horrified. Her eyes grew round in shock and anger. "I hate your chickens!"

Thea laughed all the way to the house. If she had looked over her shoulder, she would have seen Maggie pitching rocks, thick and fast, at her prized hens.

When Thea Andersen and her three children took up residence next door, Stanley and Bessie Fiske kept watch as they could see right from the beginning things were not quite right. Over the years, the path between the two homes was regularly used by Dorie, Hal, and Maggie as they eagerly found excuses to visit the neighbors. The door was always open to them and usually, there was a little something to eat.

COME TO MAMA!

Hal was the same age as Bobby Fiske. The boys were friends at school and friends at home, spending as much time together as they could manage. Hal was a clown and Bobby was the opposite. He was quiet and thoughtful. There was a bit of a melancholy around him that Hal didn't understand. The way it looked from Hal's side of the fence, his friend had everything, including loving, kind parents and a well-kept farm. In contrast, Hal came from a run-down, shabby place he was ashamed of, and he had only one parent, and she was a miserable one at that. Hal didn't know much about Bobby's early issues but he knew enough to make no mention of it. If he had asked, Bessie would have been pleased to share the details.

When her second son was born, his hearty cry brought tears of joy to his mother, as she lay waiting for him to be placed in her arms. She had predicted he would be another boy and had chosen a proper and traditional name, months before she saw him. He would be christened "Robert John" after Stanley's father and hers, a boy who would walk worthy of his grandfathers' names.

She decreed he would not be a "Bob" or any shortened version of the name. They would print "Robert" on the Saskatchewan Birth Registration, and Robert he would remain!

The attending nurse was one who never got over the wonder of a safe delivery. She excitedly proclaimed, "It's a boy!" and Bessie nodded knowingly because she already knew.

As the baby wailed his greeting to the world, Bessie noted a passing look of shock on Dr. Marshall's face. This man knew Bessie Fiske to be a woman of strength and strong character. He paused a moment as he motioned the nurse beside him to swaddle the squalling infant in a waiting blanket. The jubilant air in the room dried up, replaced by palpable tension. Though not a word had been spoken, Bessie knew something was wrong with her baby.

The doctor rested the bundle in the crook of his left arm and performed a quick, primitive examination. He placed his littlest finger in the baby's mouth and swiped upwards. Thank heavens! He felt a solid roof in the little mouth. No cleft palate. He was sure of that. Quick thoughts were going through his mind. He knew this family well. Stanley and Bessie had waited many years for little Fred, and now a brother for him was the icing on the cake. He looked at mother and baby, knowing well that she would muster strength enough for the two of them.

It is a shock for parents when they first see a child with a visible defect. Some immediately go into stages of grief - anger, denial, sorrow, and eventually (hopefully), acceptance.

"Well Bessie, we have an issue here, but you, of all people, will find a way through it."

Dr. Marshall turned the baby towards his mother and spoke in his practiced, matter-of-fact doctor voice. "This little lad has a cleft lip." In no way was Bessie expecting the wide, gaping space from her baby's left nostril, clear down to his bottom lip. The sight caused her to gasp just once. Her next words were loud and spoken with passion, as she reached for him with both arms. "Oh Bobby, come to Mama."

Forget the doctor, forget the nurse, forget the unnatural hole in her baby's face. Bessie, at that moment, was simply a mother reaching for her little one, already loving him unconditionally. The doctor was absolutely right. Bessie Fiske would see this baby through the stormy weather ahead. She looked first at the doctor and then at the nurse, and nodded her acceptance of the situation.

Stanley came. His soft heart melted when he first saw the boy, and he broke down in tears.

"Stanley, don't pity him," Bessie said defensively.

"Oh, I won't pity him, Love. It's not that. I already feel such admiration for the brave and strong lad he will be."

When Dr. Marshall came to talk to them, he was relieved to see the couple comfortably awaiting his visit. The baby was asleep in Stanley's arms and Bessie's hand, reaching from the bed, rested on the baby's blanket.

"Congratulations on another boy!" Dr. Marshall exclaimed with enthusiasm. They nodded soberly. "As to the cleft lip, it is a big concern, but the good news is, we can fix it. I have done this surgery on several babies, with favorable results." The next hour was spent with the doctor sharing his knowledge about the condition and answering their questions.

"There is no sign of a cleft palate, thankfully, which is when there is no roof in the mouth. That can be a severe complication, as it affects eating. The milk goes in, but comes out through the nose. There are also common occurrences of ear infections, speech impediments, and serious operations. As near as I can tell right now, the challenge with your baby will simply be to help him eat until we can do surgery. We will aim for about three months from now. I had time this afternoon to do a thorough exam. He does not have a cleft gum, which is also in his favor."

The doctor did not skirt around the downsides. "There will be a scar, but I will do my utmost to minimize it. There are different methods of stitching these days." He explained the intricacies of his preferred style of surgery.

"It may leave a little of what is called the "cupid's bow" effect, so there is a slight appearance of a smile. It is not disfiguring and seems to leave the least deformity. I am satisfied with the work I have done with other patients. We will have to wait to find out whether he will have issues with his teeth as time goes on. We can work on speech if it is affected. He will need reassurance from his family as he grows older. Children born with a cleft lip can be the target of cruel bullying and teasing."

The good doctor also warned them not to use the term "hare lip". "This boy is a person, not a rabbit. Call it a cleft lip and teach your friends and neighbors to do the same."

"It's a lot to consider," Stanley commented, looking down at the peaceful bundle in his arms. Stanley was a big man. In contrast, the baby looked extremely small and vulnerable.

"It's only a day at a time, folks. This could have been so much worse. This boy can live a normal life, and I will be here to support you."

This comforting conversation with the doctor would be remembered for years to come. Little Bobby Fiske had made his debut, and his parents would help him reach whatever his heart desired in the future.

Before putting on his felt hat to leave, Stanley kissed Bessie on the forehead, and the baby on his cheek. Tears were there again, shining in his eyes, as he left. Over his shoulder he said, "We'll make him the happiest kid in Saskatchewan."

Bobby was loved before he was born, and even more so after. Six-year-old Fred was thrilled to have a brother. Bessie soon adjusted to expressing breast milk and taking copious amounts of time to feed it to her thriving son. The baby's sucking ability was weak, and so she cut an "x" in the bottle nipple which allowed the milk to run out easily. At first, she had to shape his mouth around the bottle nipple and hold his lips in place with her fingers. There is a profound bonding that takes place when we interact with another human on a survival level. Patience and time resulted in satisfactory feedings and the boy grew as a Fiske baby would be expected to. Both Fred and Bobby were fine specimens, strong and hardy.

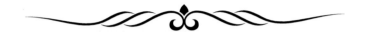

BOBBY'S JOURNEY

As predicted, Dr. Marshall performed successful surgery on Bobby's cleft lip when he was three months old. The boy was serious by nature and it took an effort to get a baby giggle out of him as he grew and explored the world around him. He did fine at school, and in those first years, he seemed oblivious to his scar and his mispronunciation of some problem words.

As he grew older though, he covered his mouth with his hands, an obvious sign he had become self-conscious. This further muffled his speech and it became an issue, especially at school.

The summer Bobby was 13, Stanley arranged to take him back to see Dr. Marshall only three months after his annual checkup. This new development of covering his face was a grave concern. Dr. Marshall reminded Stanley he had predicted Bobby may have trouble with self-esteem as he grew aware of other children's reactions.

"This is not uncommon. Find something that suits him - something he's interested in. We need to direct him toward a positive interest to take his mind off his differences, and to build his self-worth."

That's when Bobby's woodshop came into being. He had a talent for building things from wood, and he was naturally gifted at carving, even at a young age. Martin's Hardware Store in town was able to order basswood from Manitoba, known as a top-notch carving wood.

An old shed near the garden was transformed into Bobby's woodshop. They installed a window on either side so the breeze blew through, and as a bonus, it became a place to sleep on hot summer nights. Stanley added shelving and a cupboard for wood and tools. It was a well-organized hideaway for the boy to call his own.

It seemed the doctor's suggestion was working, and Bobby cheered up considerably. He and Hal spent hours together making things in the woodshop, working for Stanley, and occasionally helping Thea's hired man. Always, they landed at Bessie's table at mealtimes.

NOTHING TO SAY

Maggie stopped talking in 1942, the summer she turned nine. When Dorie came home from town for the weekend on the second Friday in September, she was struck by the change. Her little sister was distant, indifferent, and silent. No longer was she the curious pest, peeking around corners and snooping in her big sister's little suitcase.

Dorie usually paid her no attention, but now curiosity got the best of her. What was going on? All her questions were met with a shrug of Maggie's skinny shoulders, and a faraway glance towards the road. There were some gestures, pointing and staring, but no words. The little brat must be up to some new tricks, but she was taking it to the extreme. Several times when Dorie smiled at her, she simply made a face and ran away.

Thea was peeling potatoes at the sink in the kitchen when Dorie asked, "So what's up with Maggie? She won't talk."

"Attention."

"I think it's more than that, Maw. She's different."

"Always has been."

They left it at that. At suppertime, Hal came home from working at Fiske's and washed up, before taking his place at the table.

Dorie went to the door and yelled, "Come and get it!" She didn't know where the hired man was, and she mainly made the call so her little sister knew it was time to eat.

The three of them were well into the meal when the screen door opened, and Maggie burst inside. She sat at the table, grabbed some bread, and gnawed on it, careful not to look directly at any of them. Dorie felt an unfamiliar surge of warm feelings for her sister who suddenly seemed to be very alone and detached, beyond her usual quirky issues.

"What you been up to, Maggie?"

Maggie was alert, turning her head from side to side, as if she were listening for someone else to speak to her. The moment was not lost on any of them. Hal leaned toward her, offering the blue Pyrex bowl of mashed potatoes. Maggie ignored him totally, starting into another thick slice of homemade bread without butter.

Thea let out a loud breath. "Just ignore her; she's trying to get my goat. Nothing to do with you two."

And so the meal continued. There was fried chicken and Thea had made dessert, trying to lay out a special meal since Dorie was home for the first time from her boarding place in town. Two pies were waiting on the hoosier, one saskatoon, and the other raspberry. Dorie served dessert and placed the first piece of pie on Maggie's unused plate.

"I know you like raspberry best," she said, bending to look into the girl's face.

Her sister turned her head to the side, still appearing to listen intently for something far away. She ignored the pie, and after a few seconds, ran out the door.

"What the heck?" It was Hal. "When did this start?"

"All week," Thea answered. "And in case you didn't notice, she's having a heyday trying it out on you two tonight."

For some reason, Dorie, tough Dorie, felt her voice quaver as she said, "Maw, I don't like it. Did you do anything to her?"

Thea turned her back to them as she left the table, carrying the dirty plates and setting them in the sink. "Of course I didn't do anything to her. You know I can't make her behave. She does whatever she friggin' well wants to."

The conversation abruptly ended as Riley, the hired man came in, and washed his hands in the small basin on a wooden stand near the door. He was late because he had been working in the north field and it was a long drive on the tractor to get back to the house. He helped himself to a full plate and grinned as he topped the whole meal with gravy.

"This looks swell!" He sat at the table and discussed with Hal their plans to mow the hayfield and sharpen the mower blade. Dorie poured hot water from the kettle on the stove into the sink for dishwashing.

"Do you want to do the dishes together, Maw, or would you like a break?"

Thea answered with a shrug, "Don't matter." But obviously, she preferred the break, as she went out the door. Dorie could see her through the window as she settled on the wooden chair out on the porch. Her wild red hair was streaked with grey, and her brown dress was faded and wrinkled.

Unconcerned about Riley listening, Dorie approached the table, gathering up the remaining dishes.

"Come on you guys, I've been away all week but you've been here. Something's going on."

Riley took a minute to swallow and then said, "The little one seems to have quit talking, and she's jumpy. Is that what you mean?"

"Yeah, that's what I mean all right. Hal, what do you think?"

"I dunno. I hardly saw her. I have been working for Stanley all week."

"Does Maw know something she's not telling?"

Hal shrugged. "Who knows?"

Dorie grinned at Riley. "Crazy family you're working for!"

"Oh, I've seen crazier."

Riley was about 30, and he seemed to be a drifter. Thea had recently hired him. He didn't talk about where he came from or where he was going. He had hired on a couple of weeks before, for haying and harvest.

"I mind my own business", he added, as he continued with his pie, his fork chasing the saskatoons that were rolling out of the crust.

"And just so you know, I don't judge the people I work for. I won't be saying anything to anybody about whatever goes on here."

"Sometimes it gets bad," Dorie said honestly, not trying to hide anything from Riley who was still a stranger to them. She worried now that she was in town. She worried for her sister.

The men left the house and Dorie finished up the dishes. When she went outside to where her mother had been sitting, she saw only the empty kitchen chair. She could see Thea carrying two pails of water from the well to the chicken run, which was surrounded by four-foot-high chicken wire. Her shoulders rocked from side to side as she made her way towards the henhouse.

"The chickens are Maw's happy place," Dorie said aloud, to no one in particular. She watched Thea lift the heavy pails of water, and fill the drinking containers in the pen.

Dorie surveyed the farmyard and conceded this wasn't much of a place to come home to. Living in town was even better than she had imagined. After only two weeks away, she was ready to leave the farm for good.

For Dorie, it was a brand-new life, with interesting people, and a fresh start in school. She boarded with two girls from farms outside town. The three of them went for walks in the evenings on the sidewalks, which she liked better than the dirt paths around the farm. The scenery was better, too. As they walked around town after supper, they often caught the eye of some of the boys who played scrub at the ball diamond beside the school. Dorie felt fortunate to fit in so quickly to her current surroundings.

The three girls from the boarding place were inseparable. The tall one, Muriel, was always cracking jokes and had a knack for helping them settle into living away from home. Jean was a plain Jane type, but smart as a whip, and eager to help the other two with their school work.

Dorie noticed Maggie making her way across the road to Fiske's. She wondered if they ever got tired of her snooping around their place. Should she go tell them to send her home when they wanted to? Dorie pondered this unusual development. Why wouldn't Maggie talk? Her strange behavior was puzzling.

CAN YOU MAKE HER TALK?

Stanley was pleased they had made progress with Bobby's issues by the time he was 13. Dr. Marshall's advice to pursue a special interest had worked wonders! He was now one year older, and turning out some excellent wood pieces to sell. Hal was the salesman of the two and they schemed how to market their wares.

At this point, Maggie was ten and she had not spoken for over a year, except for a few scant words which were reserved for Bessie and Stanley. Their silent, young neighbor was on their minds all summer.

Finally, Stanley persuaded Thea to take Maggie to the same doctor who had been so helpful to Bobby over the years since his initial surgery. She resisted at first until Stanley volunteered to provide a ride for the two of them. He even offered to make the appointment. A couple of weeks later, on a hot afternoon, he drove into Thea's yard to pick them up. He had some misgivings about making the trip, although he had topped up the radiator with water before he left. If the truck conked out on the way, he believed he could tinker with it enough to get it back on the road.

Stanley had promised Maggie candy on the ride home after the appointment. He admitted to Bessie that it was a bribe, but otherwise there was a real possibility she may run out of the doctor's office and down the street!

Always the careful sort, Stanley warned Thea as they were about to head out. "Don't lean on that door. It could fly open."

Maggie was sitting between them, avoiding the large gear shift that was taking up the space right in front of her. A wide grin spread across her face. Stanley knew she was imagining the possible catastrophe he had just mentioned to her mother.

There was not much conversation to be had. The sound of the truck motor was loud, giving off a low growl along with a high, whistling sound. It worried Stanley as they covered the dusty miles.

"Not long till we get the candy," he said, looking at Maggie. No comment from either of his passengers.

The doctor was older than Stanley and had become a friend since he operated on Bobby's cleft lip. During the past fourteen years, Stanley had been in this office countless times. He was pleased to see the doctor immediately referred Thea and Maggie to his nurse. She was the one who had been so helpful regarding Bobby's speech. Stanley told them he would be waiting in the truck.

Thea was less than cooperative. She and Maggie were led into another room with high windows and very tall ceilings. Three chairs were set fairly close together. As the nurse took her seat, she cheerfully invited Thea and Maggie to make themselves comfortable. The nurse had a small notebook and an Eversharp pencil, and was ready to begin collecting information. Maggie appeared to be listening for some far-off sound, often turning her head towards the windows. She had become quite proficient at this acting, as she raised her eyes to the ceiling and made like she was deeply concentrating.

Thea filled the chair, with a little overhang on each side, and she crossed her arms over her ample bosom. She wore the green and white dress Dorie had chosen from the catalog for Fred Fiske's wedding. Fred's wedding had been postponed until the following year because the farm he had planned to rent was not available until then. He and Colleen would have to wait. Dorie insisted Thea wear the new dress to the doctor's appointment, as she knew her mother didn't have anything decent enough to wear to the city, except for it. Besides, Fred might cancel again. Maybe he just had cold feet. It wouldn't hurt for Thea to wear it now and then.

Maggie, too, was wearing a dress that day, the one they had bought for the same occasion. It was yellow and somehow not the best color for her. The skirt came just above her knees and if anyone was taking notice, they would have seen dark lines across the back of her legs. Her summer souvenir. She insisted on wearing the pointy-toed, brown boots Hal had bought for a dollar at the store in town.

They looked rather odd with the dress, especially on such a hot day, but truth be told, both Stanley and Thea were pleased she didn't push to go barefoot.

The nurse, Florence (well-named for a nurse), was tall and thin, with a white belted dress that had been starched almost to death. Stanley had no doubt that if he got Thea and Maggie there, he could count on Florence to do the rest. She had been their angel in dealing with Bobby, helping him with his speech, forming certain sounds that were once impossible for him, building confidence, and helping him overcome his tendency to cover his mouth with his hand. Her knowledge had smoothed out so many practical details, improving the boy's skills and attitude.

Sitting in the hot room, Florence realized she had a bigger challenge before her than she'd had with Bobby Fiske many years ago. The Andersens appeared not to be looking for answers, as Stanley and Bessie had. They had been desperate to do whatever it took to give their son a normal life. Florence suspected Thea's hesitancy was due to the unfamiliar setting, and that underneath her sour demeanor, she was concerned about her silent daughter.

The nurse had peroxide blonde, wavy hair, white duty shoes, and those white nurse stockings that must have been hot as a firecracker. Her well-lipsticked, rosebud mouth fascinated Maggie as she stared intently to observe what words would come out.

"Well, let's begin." Florence tried to sound chipper, but the atmosphere was uncomfortable.

"I'm Florence. I'll need a little information to start." Thea was stone-faced and Maggie was listening for her imaginary sounds, turning her ear to the open screened window.

Florence dived right in, "And when did this girl stop talking?"

The question could have been directed at either of them. Maggie filled her cheeks with air and held her lips tightly together. She shrugged her shoulders as if she'd never heard of such a thing as not talking. Thea, by now, appeared to be feeling the heat of an expected answer and shrugged her shoulders as well.

She answered briefly, "While ago."

The girl knew exactly when she stopped talking. It was the day she got switched three times in a row, or almost, for making ugly faces at her mother.

After two switchings (the second one much more vicious than the first), Maggie stepped closer to Thea and defiantly stuck out her tongue. Dorie, forever preoccupied with herself and her looks, had perfected the art of shutting out her surroundings and the mayhem that often took over their home. On this particular day, she had been listening from the living room, and suddenly she was right there, between her sister and her mother. Thea had already grabbed her stick for a third round, but Dorie stood in front of her, spreading her arms on both sides, guarding her sister.

"Don't you touch her again, Maw. Don't you dare."

And then, Dorie, the self-appointed referee, turned to Maggie to finally settle the issue. She looked directly into Maggie's rebellious little face, contorted with anger and pain, eyes brimming.

"And Maggie," she ordered, you can make ugly faces at her all you want to, but turn away from her when you do it. Don't let her see it." The mandated truce had worked. From then on several times a day, the girl swiveled her head around to hide her face from her mother. Thea knew exactly what was going on, but even though Dorie moved to town to go to school, her warning had taken effect.

Of course, none of this was reported to the sweet and kindly nurse who tried yet another approach. "I know your neighbors, Mr. and Mrs. Fiske. In fact, I know them very well. As you are probably aware, Bobby was our patient here."

Maggie suddenly was all ears, finally showing interest in the here and now, instead of cocking her head to hear imaginary messages. She nodded at the mention of the Fiske family.

"I hear that you sometimes talk to them but to no one else, is that right, Maggie?"

The child puffed her cheeks with air again. It was a novel trick she had practiced the night before, in front of the mirror in her upstairs bedroom. She had decided it looked even better when she squeezed her eyes shut at the same time.

Florence, patient as a nurse should be, turned to Thea and said kindly, "Mrs. Anderson, how can I help?"

"Can you make her talk?"

Florence was calm and unfazed, no doubt a technique taught in her nursing classes years before.

"Well, Mrs. Andersen, the fact is, Maggie *can* talk. We already know that, but believe it or not, it's hard for her to speak. It is almost impossible in most situations."

"Humph!" It was an audible grunt of derision from Thea.

Maggie had begun to wink quickly, first with one eye and then with the other, over and over, back and forth, left to right. She had practiced that, too. The atmosphere was strained. Maggie's shenanigans triggered a bit of a chuckle from Florence, and she coughed as she tried to suppress it.

"You know, Miss Maggie, I think you and I just might get along!"

There was another grunt from Thea as she heaved herself out of her chair and smoothed the clammy green skirt of her dress. Without a word, she lumbered to the door and went out.

Florence waited a few seconds. "So now Maggie, what do you have to say?" The furious winking resumed.

"I know a little about children who have difficulty talking. I'd like to tell you about it and I am sure you will find it interesting."

Maggie was again listening for sounds outside the window. "In your case, Maggie, you *can* talk. You talk to Stanley and Bessie Fiske because you feel safe with them. I contacted your school teacher and she said you sometimes whisper to her. When you don't practice talking at all, it gets easier and easier to just stay quiet."

The nurse continued, although she felt like she was speaking to a distracted flurry of nonsensical blinks and puffy cheeks.

"Without using words, people only know a part of who you are. Do you know that your voice is really important? You can use your words to be a good friend, a good sister, even a good daughter." Maggie's face belied her feelings. The mention of "daughter" brought on a dark look.

"Is it easier for you not to talk at all, Maggie?" The girl nodded.

"Does what I'm telling you make sense?"

Maggie shook her head, and just then, as if she remembered the promised candy, she ran out the door, hot on the heels of her mother.

Nurse Florence sat for a few moments in her chair by the window, shaking her head. Elective mutism was a fascinating topic with more questions than answers. This was a tough case. She had a feeling she would not see this pair again.

Despite Stanley's worries, the old truck made it not only to the gas station on the way out of town, where they filled the tank and bought some hard candy for Maggie, but it got them safely home. On the way, Maggie sucked on a large striped piece of candy as she practiced her new found facial grimacing. She puffed up her cheeks and sealed her lips. She knew she was improving at it, and seemed to be amused to no end with herself. Thea sat well away from the door due to Stanley's warning that she could fall out. She looked out the window as they rode home, and Stanley assumed she was mad about how the appointment had gone.

The man was a strong believer in communication. "Well Thea, I take it you walked out on the nurse?"

Something like a snort came from her corner of the cab, followed by her brief explanation. "Waste-a-time."

"Well, I knew it was a longshot, but I figured it was worth a try."

There was no further comment. Stanley persevered as patiently as if he were nurse Florence herself. He continued to speak as if they were having a normal conversation.

"You know, a person has to keep on trying different ways to solve a problem. We wrangled over Bobby's troubles over and over, from Day One."

No response. Stanley was determined to make use of the opportunity to converse. He carried on amiably.

"She helped Bobby and that's why I wanted you to at least meet Florence." Thea's arms were folded over her belly, flattening her bosom.

"Hah! Didn't do him much good. He still sounds like a snarf."

Stanley's head whipped to the side as he took his eyes off the road and stared in disbelief at this rude and ungrateful woman. The

Fiske men had the curse of going beet red in the face when they were mad. Fred had it too, as well as Bobby. Stanley's face was nearly purple as he worked his jaw. Level-headed and slow to get mad - that was Stanley Fiske.

Silence reigned. Her cruel words had cut him down. The truck pulled up beside the Andersen's house, and Thea shoved a crumpled five-dollar bill at Maggie, motioning with her head towards their driver. Maggie looked bewildered. She held up the bill in the space between the two adults. Stanley had not uttered a word since Thea's insult.

"Not a chance, Woman. Keep your money!"

The passengers got out. Thea hoisted herself off the sticky seat, and Maggie slid across to the door and got out, just before her mother slammed it shut. The old truck roared out of the yard and by the way it swerved onto the road, Maggie knew Stanley Fiske was boiling over. That night after dark, Hal was dispatched to the Fiske's back porch where he left a wooden egg crate, filled to the top with 12 dozen eggs.

THE BIG CLOCK

The Big Clock first entered Maggie's imagination during her silent years. One Saturday afternoon, she watched Bessie carefully clean the wind-up chime clock that stood on the buffet in the Fiske farmhouse. It was an ornate piece with carved leaf designs around the edges, and a fascinating little door on the front. Bessie took special care, oiling the hinges and the moving parts of the clock. Maggie watched with wide eyes, especially intrigued with the gears that met with precision. She watched intently as even the key was polished, along with the gold-colored pendulum. Maggie had been taught to tell time at school and she also understood the Roman numerals on the face of the clock. She had just passed into Grade 4 and even though some of the work was hard, she had quickly caught on to telling time - the hours, the minutes, and the seconds as they ticked by.

In her mind, she saw another clock, as big as a house. It was a monstrosity, and she could take a look at it any time she wanted to. She could watch as it precisely marked off the March of Time around the world.

The teacher at Aroma School had explained the different time zones to her students. That was hard to understand, but she said time was carefully calculated in every country of the world, according to the sun. The Big Clock often came to Maggie's childish mind. It marked the day she was born, the day she stopped talking, anything special or even not so special. Her birthday shone bright gold when she thought of the clock. It was marked by ten bright and sparkling jewels, one for each year, beside the date: June 10, 1933. Her birthday was never noticed at home, but the teacher wrote: "Happy Birthday,

Maggie" on the blackboard way up in the corner. She did the same when other students had a birthday.

Maggie decided the Big Clock was not her friend. She did not like its face. Occasionally, Bessie asked Stanley to adjust their wind-up chime clock because the timing was off. Sometimes the Big Clock's timing was off, too - way off! Or, maybe it was only a smidge off and caused people to miss out on something special, just by a hair. Did Maggie barely miss out on having a dad? Did she miss him by mere minutes, or by years?

The girl had an inquisitive mind, but did not share her unusual questions with anyone, and so there were few answers. Additional odd thoughts possessed her thinking, but the Big Clock consistently came to mind to give her pause for thought.

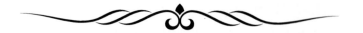

TRAINING CHICKENS

Bessie was concerned that Maggie's silence continued as the summer weeks passed. The appointment with Dr. Marshall and Nurse Florence had rendered no solution whatsoever.

Bessie decided to act on an idea she had been working on ever since the ill-fated appointment. Dandelions were overpowering the daisies and pansies that volunteered their presence around the yard. The place had never looked this poor for years. Bessie had wished for renewed energy all summer to keep up the yard and the garden.

Talking out loud as was her habit, Bessie declared her intention. "If Maggie isn't willing to learn to cook, I'll take her on as my chief gardener and yard keeper!" She started across the field to the farm next door. She decided to talk to Thea about hiring young Maggie for a summer job.

Bessie's boys often teased her about her conversations with herself. Sometimes they sneaked up on her to listen in and then would interject a comment.

"Go on with you!" was her customary response, and her ready laugh was what the boys were aiming for. It was close to a cackle if she found something really funny. Stanley once told the boys, "When Mama's happy, we're all happy!"

Bessie knew Maggie was lonely and she felt sorry for her. Maybe the idea of yard work would work out for both of them. Maggie noticed Bessie's approach even before she got to the gate. Not taught in the graces of sociable conversation, Maggie ran to meet Bessie, looked her in the eye, and asked, "What?"

It was remarkable the girl spoke occasionally to both Stanley and Bessie, but not to others. She was no chatterbox, but if they were alone, she sometimes chose to say a few words.

Bessie replied, "I came to talk to your mother about you doing some work for me. What do you think of that?"

A doubtful smirk spread across Maggie's freckles. As she stepped ahead of Bessie to lead the way to the house, Bessie was horrified to see raised red welts across the back of the skinny legs. She reached for Maggie's hand and turned her around.

"Did she do that to you?"

Maggie nodded, matter-of-factly. She then suddenly began to talk, as freely as Bessie had ever heard her speak.

"She said to put on overalls to hide the marks, but I didn't. It's too hot."

"When did she do it?"

"Last night."

Bessie was aware of Thea watching them as they conversed near the porch.

"Why did she do such a thing?"

Again, Bessie detected a slight smirk as Maggie answered, "I was training her chickens." Bessie was silent, trying to suppress her indignation. The many welts were deep and ugly. They would last for a long time. Maggie came up with an excuse, lest Bessie would also be angry about the chickens.

"I *was* training them."

The older woman found her voice. She asked incredulously, "However would you train a chicken?"

"Well... exercise."

Bessie stifled a smile, and still holding the girl's hand, she turned back towards her own house.

Maggie motioned towards the house as if to ask, "You don't want to talk to her?"

Bessie had picked up the pace. They left the yard in a hurry. "Not just now. I might say too much!"

Thea was washing dishes at the kitchen sink. If she had been prone to talk out loud as Bessie did, she would have said something like, "Tattletale brat!"

And so it was that Maggie learned the joys of gardening. Her young energy was just what Bessie needed to restore the yard, and

Maggie thrived as she escaped much of the lonely summer, no longer captive to her mother's moods throughout the long days.

She was Bessie's right hand - watering, weeding, and killing dandelions. They avoided the afternoon heat, working in the mornings and again, later in the day. As the yard and vegetable garden took shape under Bessie's direction and Maggie's eager hands, the flowers bloomed in profusion.

Three weeks after Maggie started yard work, Bessie stood on the step and called Maggie from the garden. Tall, yellow daylilies waved in the light breeze beside them. Bessie and Maggie sat together on the step and surveyed the yard.

"Just look at what you've done here, Maggie! Things are looking shipshape."

Maggie nodded, well pleased with the accomplishment and the praise. Bessie opened her small leather change purse. It had a clasp that was hard to open and closed with a loud snap.

"Today is payday, young lady."

She held out two quarters and did not expect the response that erupted. Maggie snatched the coins from Bessie's outstretched palm and threw them in the dirt by the step. Before she ran, she whispered, "I don't like money. I like flowers."

Bessie left the money where it was. She was a fairly heavy-set lady and retrieving it would not have been easy. Bobby could fetch it later, or as Bessie said aloud to herself, "Maggie may think better of it, and come back for it herself."

The Fiskes later learned the details of the chicken training that had gone on next door. Stanley came in at 3 o'clock for a drink of water and a snack. Maggie was in the house, waiting with Bessie for the heat in the garden to let up. Stanley leaned back in his chair at the head of the table.

"So I hear you've taken to training the chickens."

Maggie smiled, and then confessed, "I can't do it anymore."

Stanley nodded. "From what I heard, that's probably best." Maggie noticed the red sweat mark across his forehead from his felt hat. She stared at him, as if deciding whether or not to speak. They had learned that she might talk if they didn't rush her or appear to be too interested.

After a long delay, two or three minutes at least, she volunteered, "Hal bought me pointy-toed, boots in town. They cost a buck."

Stanley nodded. He remembered she wore them when they went to Stillwater to see the doctor.

"They're the best for chasing chickens. I ran in the pen to rile them up." The look on her face showed she relished the memory of it. "They were flying right off the ground, up in air, crocking..."

"Crocking?"

"Yeah, that's the sound when they're riled."

No one spoke for a while.

Maggie started up the conversation again, grinning as she said, "Their feathers were floating in the air, and some hens went right out a little hole under the wire."

"Oh, no!" That was Bessie, egging her on.

Maggie looked out the window. "Dumb chickens! You know we got that hawk."

For lack of knowing what to say, but hoping to keep the girl talking, Stanley remarked, "Poor old hens!"

Maggie squinted her eyes, mentally reviewing the scene. She said to no one in particular, appearing like Bessie when she talked to herself.

"It was fun." She nodded her head as if to convince her listeners. "A lot of fun."

The old folks managed to contain themselves, but later that evening, sitting on the porch in the cool of the evening before bed, they told Bobby and Fred the story of the pointy-toed, brown boots. Bessie laughed till tears rolled down her cheeks. "Exercise! Just exercise and training!"

RESCUED AGAIN

The summer passed quickly, and the school bell rang once again. Who do you suppose should show their ugly faces at the school door on that first day back! Bobby and Hal were disgusted to see Oliver Meyer was back, with Sam Holmes by his side, both sneering at them as they went in the door to put their lunches on the cloakroom shelf

The bullies were back in fine form. Once again, "Maggie Rooster" became the word of the day. And then, they turned their insults in another direction.

Hal and Bobby asked the teacher if they could use the ball and a couple of flat, leather ball gloves from the ball bag in the basement of the school. When she agreed, they headed to the ball diamond to finish off the noon hour with a game of catch. Sam and Oliver were waiting for them at the backstop.

Oliver, still the leader of the pair, looked at Bobby with a sneer. "We got a new name for you. We're gonna call you 'Kisser'. With that mug of yours, you'd be real slick at it."

Sam piped up, "But who'd wanna kiss *that!*" The boys had rehearsed their lines and laughed raucously. It was fake laughing, and they were doing it for dirtiness. When the bell rang and the students found their way back into the school, Bobby was missing. The teacher asked if anyone had seen him. No one said anything.

Oliver was feeling his oats. "Ask little Maggie Rooster there. She knows a lot about the Fiskes." Of course, everyone knew there was no point in asking Maggie anything. She didn't speak. The young teacher had big trouble on her hands. She already had the challenge of a mute student, and now the two bullies were pushing her. She didn't have a clue how to handle them.

40

Suddenly, the open door at the back of the room filled with the body of a tall and angry man. It was Fred Fiske, back again. He tipped his hat to Miss Newberry, and said, "Excuse me, ma'am." He dragged Oliver and Sam out of their desks. As the students sat in their seats, they could hear yelling and bawling going on outside, and they could hear every word of Fred's deep and threatening voice.

"I thought we settled this last year. I can come here every day until you straighten up, or you can drop out and not bother coming back. Either way, I won't be far away." They all heard Fred's truck leave the schoolyard. Bobby walked in and took his seat, his eyes burning with anger. His tormentors disappeared for the afternoon.

The next day Sam came alone, subdued and with his head down. He managed to catch a moment with Maggie on the school steps as the bell rang at 9.

"Sorry, Maggie. You won't hear it again." For anyone watching closely, they may have caught a glimpse of Ben Holmes standing at the edge of the trees that surrounded the schoolyard. He would keep his son in line, whatever it took.

It appeared that Oliver had dropped out, as Fred strongly suggested. The days at school took on a better atmosphere. The teacher let down her guard and found ways to loosen the reins and allow the children to enjoy their learning.

Bobby was gaining back his confidence, now that Oliver was out of the picture. He and Hal were big-hearted enough to treat Sam decently. Thousands may not have, but Bobby had been brought up right, and Hal knew enough to follow suit.

SUMMER OF GOODBYE

Spring came as always. The birds returned from wintering in the South. The first to arrive were the crows, and their caw-caw-ing sound was a welcome sign that winter was over. Soon after, the snow melted, and purple crocuses bloomed close to the ground on the hill behind the school. Fuzzy, grey pussy willows appeared on the poplar trees. By the middle of May, they had been replaced with the greenest of spring leaves. The youngest students at school talked about the baby calves at their farm and batches of kittens. Spring was in the air, and was an ample reward to all for enduring the long winter.

Most of the Grade 8 students were buckling down to study for exams at the end of June. They would have to go to the bigger school in town to write the exams and be supervised there. They were feeling the pressure.

Every one of them would be leaving Aroma School. A few would go on to school in town for Grade 9, but for most their school days would be over, and their lives would change forever. Maggie wondered if Hal would work the farm so his mother wouldn't have to hire someone as she always had. Maggie wondered and listened, but of course, she couldn't ask.

It was Stanley who decided Bobby would go to town school. "He's not a farmer like Fred. I understand the land is not for everyone. I think another year of school will give the boy time to make up his mind about what he wants to do. Education is always an important thing."

School in the fall would be different for Maggie. For the first time, she would walk to school alone. That was the problem with being the youngest. There was always that feeling of being left behind.

On the way home from school, on June 30th, Hal announced to Maggie and Bobby he had made his decision. His school days were over. Thea told him it was his choice to continue his schooling in town as his sister was doing, or he could quit. He lost no time grabbing his dream of freedom.

When Bobby asked if he would work the farm for his mother, Hal answered, "Not in a million years!" He said he had some ideas about a job where he could make an easy buck one way or another. He was of age to quit. Thea applied no pressure on her son to stay in school, as Stanley Fiske did on his.

Hal was in a high mood, basking in the knowledge that his school career had come to a glorious end. Grandstanding as always, Hal ran ahead of the other two and then turned so he was walking backward, talking to them, until they caught up.

"*No more school days, No more books, No more teacher's dirty looks!*" He chanted the childish words that umpteen students repeated on the last day of school each year.

When neither Bobby nor Maggie paid attention to his worn-out rhyme, he said, "Hey Maggie, did you pass?"

She shrugged. As far as anyone knew, she hadn't given her report card at first glance, let alone a second. She had done the bare minimum of work at school. She wasn't expected to participate in class due to her silence, and so it had been a lonely year. She didn't take much to reading, even though her Aunt Marion from Stillwater sent a brand-new book in the mail each year for her birthday. They were popular books, perfect for her reading and interest level with titles such as *The Secret Garden, Black Beauty,* and *An Old Fashioned Girl.* Maggie had not read any of them but they were placed, one by one, on her bedroom windowsill for decoration.

For months, she had looked forward to Dorie coming home for the summer. Maybe they could be friends. Maybe Maw would be happier and Dorie might again put a stop to the switchings. Maybe. As it turned out, Dorie did come, but she stayed only three days. She got bad news right after she arrived, and said she couldn't stand it at home another minute. So she went back to town to her same boarding place. The lady there planned to board road construction workers for the summer and she hired Dorie to help in the kitchen.

The dreadful news she received was about her friend Muriel, the fun-loving one she had lived with during the school months for the past two years. She was the girl with sparkling eyes and a perpetual hint of a smile on her face. She was always telling jokes and making life better for the other girls, especially when they first adjusted to town school. Muriel came to the chicken farm for a short visit one Saturday a few weeks before. She took a special interest in Maggie and gave her a kerchief with blue paisley designs on it.

She talked openly to Maggie about her silence. "Dorie tells me you can't talk just now, but that you will sometime soon. When that day comes, we'll have a dandy old visit." She put her arm around Maggie's thin shoulders. The girl was starved for love and wished Muriel was her sister instead of Dorie.

The saddest news was that Muriel had been riding in the front seat of the family car, between her mother and father. A big logging truck was directly in front of them, and when the driver slammed on his brakes, a loose pole from his load shot backward, straight towards their car. It shattered the windshield and pierced her chest. She was in the wrong place at the wrong time. A few seconds either way could have saved her, but she died. She was only sixteen years old.

The Big Clock flashed into Maggie's mind. Muriel's short years came to a screeching halt with the happen-chance of a flying log and the clanging bells of the Big Clock. Three days ago the pendulum stopped for Dorie's best friend. The Big Clock was precise and unyielding. Its steady tick-tock did not miss a second. Muriel, time to go.

A lonely summer was looming, for both Maggie and Bobby. With Hal quitting school, Bobby already worried every day over how school would go for him in the fall. He knew the taunting would assuredly come his way as before, but as Fred was getting married and moving to his own place, there would be no big brother to back him up. And unless Hal changed his mind about returning to school, Bobby would have to stand alone. This was anxiety like he had not known before.

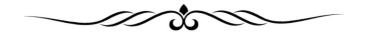

LOSING A BROTHER

Fred would be married in July, and plans were underway inside and outside the Fiske house. The welcome bride-to-be was the plump and pretty Colleen Krydor, who was eager to impress Bessie. The two women spent numerous days together as a housekeeping school of sorts unfolded. Together they stitched a quilt. Another day they hemmed flour sacks for dish towels, sewed potholders, and embroidered pillowcases. They made several items a girl would normally have collected in her hope chest, if she was lucky enough to have one. Since Colleen's family had very little to spare, the young couple was in dire need of the basics, and Bessie set out to remedy that.

She was thrilled to be getting a daughter at last. Several friends and neighbors reminded Bessie of the line, "Remember, you're not losing a son, you're gaining a daughter." It was true, and Bessie was relieved that Colleen was a pleasant girl who was eager to fit into the family. They knew her well, as she and Fred had been going steady for nearly two years.

No one tried to tell Bobby he was gaining a sister, but he felt the painful reality of "losing a brother". He felt the sting of Fred moving out. In fact, his brother had already spent a few nights over at the rented farm, seeding the crop. Even now before the wedding, Fred's mind was on the exciting path he was taking, not only his marriage but on the challenge of the rented farm.

The farmhouse there needed a lot of work. The roof leaked over the bedroom add-on, and that would have to be fixed before they could move in. The place had been occupied by an elderly bachelor who passed on, and the entire farm had been sadly neglected. The rush on the spring work was a pressure to Fred, and the machinery in the farmyard needed repair. It was old and rusty, but like his dad, Fred had a knack for mechanics. A man can do a lot with haywire and a little know-how!

The house was actually in deplorable condition. Bessie and Maggie accompanied Stanley there one morning, armed with a broom and a mop and a cream can full of hot water. The two of them did a temporary clean-up in the kitchen and one of the bedrooms. Bessie, always thrifty to a fault, actually threw out some kitchen items that she deemed too filthy to resurrect. Even hot water and soap wouldn't do much for them.

Maggie enjoyed the day, imagining the place when it would be sparkling clean and freshly painted. Bessie had packed sandwiches, and they chose to go outside to eat in the fresh air. Bessie said she could smell mice in the house. A couple of cats from the barn at home would fix that problem. Never one to sit still, Maggie explored the yard between bites of her sandwich, waving and pointing with each find.

When Bessie was finished her lunch, she joined Maggie at the various spots in the yard where irises grew in profusion. She was also pleased to see the bright red, Maltese Cross that Maggie had discovered, and a big stand of rhubarb by the lilacs. For such a young child, Maggie was surprisingly obsessed with plants, trees, and shrubs of all kinds. Near the dilapidated back steps, she found tiny, pale yellow snapdragons that must have grown smaller with each passing year. Once upon a time this yard was loved and cared for, and Maggie felt confident the young couple would restore it. She wondered if Colleen liked to work outside, or if she was more of a stay-in-the-house type.

Their hard work was not lost on the groom-to-be. When he and his dad returned to the house in the afternoon, he looked around with a grin. "It *is* going to be a home after all! I was wondering if it would ever be fit to live in."

Bessie reassured him. "Ah, this is just the beginning. We'll get Colleen over here next time and you won't believe what three women and some elbow grease can do!"

It was time for the older Fiskes to head home, but Fred would be staying another night. He stood in the doorway and yelled, "Thanks a million!" as the truck lurched and then roared out the dusty lane. As expected, Bessie left some food supplies on the table—a loaf of bread, butter and jam, and a sealer of soup.

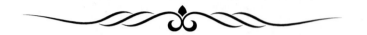

WHAT AM I BID?

Bobby was given a choice to come along to Fred's or to stay home. It was Saturday, and sometimes he and Hal went shooting gophers. Hal was the one with ideas when they were allotted free time. Preparing for June exams was not on their list.

The boys were near the road when a truck pulled over. The driver cranked the window open and asked, "Do you know the Olsen farm?"

The boys looked at each other. Bobby answered, "Yes, I've been there. Go straight ahead to the train tracks and turn west."

The man behind the wheel said, "Auction sale there, going on right now. You two want to ride along?" They didn't need to be asked twice. Hal and Bobby jumped into the truck box at the same time and stood as the truck rolled down the road. They managed to keep their balance on the short ride to the Olsen farm a few miles away.

There was something about the auction that set them a-buzz. The sale hadn't quite started yet, but people were already milling around, checking out the household items, pawing through boxes, inspecting tools, books, and all manner of fascinating junk displayed on the makeshift tables. Two auctioneers sat at a small table on the back of a wide truck box, committed to extracting every possible penny out of their day's work.

One auctioneer had a piece of paper in front of him and held a pencil in his hand. He greeted the crowd that had gathered closely around the truck.

"Good morning, Folks. We are the Higgins brothers. I'm John, and here's Ron. Pleased today to be trusted with the sale of the Olsen family goods. As some of you know, the farmland here has been sold and we'll take care of the rest. We'll start with the smaller household items, and proceed in the afternoon to the machinery beside the out-buildings over there. The truck will be moved throughout the day so you can stay close enough not to miss a sale. We'll keep things rolling and get you all home in time to milk your cows tonight."

The other brother, Ron, was bigger and wore a black cowboy hat with a red and yellow braided band. He waved and caught everyone's attention when he yelled out, "Higgins Auctioneers at your service." By now, a young teenager wearing a similar hat had grabbed a couple of items off the nearest table and held them up. Suddenly, the air was vibrating as Ron Higgins flipped into a different voice altogether.

"Selling Grandma's quilt. You've all been looking at it. And here we go. Will ya give me five dollars, five dollars, give me five dollars and go! Five dollars, now six, will ya' give me seven, six-fifty then, six-fifty, six-fifty!" The hammer hit the table. "SOLD!"

The lucky bidder looked slightly dazed but pleased to step up to pay and take his prize. The sellers kept things moving quickly. There was a sense of "buy it now" and often the words "don't lose the bid" were thrown into the mix. Something about his rhythm kept the crowd engaged.

Bobby and Hal looked on with amazement. The singsong chant of the auction excited them both. They moved in closer as the steady beat continued. If only they had a few bucks to get in on the action!

Riley tapped Hal on the shoulder and said, "Didn't know you were coming. I could have given you a ride."

Hal answered, "Didn't know I was coming either!" Riley pulled out his wallet and offered a handful of bills, mostly 1s and 2s.

"These are yours."

Hal shook his head, "Nah."

"Your mom overpaid my wages last night. Told her it was too much and she said to give the extra to you."

"Huh?"

"Said she wants you to stick around home this summer and stay out of trouble. Said it would do you good to work with me."

"Well, this money is what will do me good right now! Come on Bobby, let's buy Fred a wedding present."

The auctioneer was full of energy.

"What am I bid on this set of dishes? Pretty as a picture. Feed the whole family!" The young man holding up auction items hoisted the box of dishes onto the table and showed off a plate and a cup. They were cream-colored dishes with blue flowers in the middle of each plate.

"Here we go now, start at three. three dollar bid, now four. Four dollar bid, now five, five, four-fifty now. Yes and five dollar bid. I've got four-fifty now." The hammer came down on the table. "SOLD to the fine lookin' guy with the big smile!"

Hal stepped up to take possession of the dishes that would grace Fred and Colleen's table. Bobby wished he had some cash. He had noticed assorted household items the young couple could use, and he was in a buying mood. Riley was right beside him.

"Wanna borrow a few bucks and get in on the auction?" Bobby had never borrowed money in his life before, but he couldn't resist. The next couple of hours were fun like the boys never had before. Fred and Colleen were going to have a pile of wedding gifts come July!

The auctioneers kept at it. The boy helping them held up a flowered glass pot.

John yelled out, "Hey, a thunder mug for under the bed!"

Ron took over the selling, "Never know when you gotta go! Thunder mug, fifty cents. Don't be shy. I'm bid fifty cents, I'm bid now a dollar, dollar now, dollar now, no bids, fifty cents. Mark 'er cheap."

The men took a break at noon to have a quick bite of lunch, and then moved the truck closer to the bigger items near the house. Sitting out in the sun was an iron bedstead with springs, a round table, a rocking chair, a churn, and boxes of junk. There was a lot yet to sell.

Bobby and Hal approached John and Ron Higgins. "This is great stuff!" Hal commented with his ever-present grin. "First auction for us."

"Really? Well, boys, it is a lot of fun. It's work, yes, but we love it. We've been doing it since we were your age. Our dad got us going early on."

"How hard is it to learn?" It was still Hal doing all the talking.

John turned to Bobby and included him. "It's not hard at all. You just have to know your numbers. Count by 5s - 5, 10, 15, 20, 25. You gotta do it without thinking. Go back down the other way - 25, 20, 15, 10, 5. Practice till you can do it with your eyes shut - 10, 9,8,7,6,5,4,3,2,1. And then you throw in your fillers. Everybody finds their own extra words that feel just right for them. Ron likes to say, 'will ya give me' and he often says 'dollar bid'."

I often say, "I'm bid at one now, I'm bid at two now, I'm bid at three now. Of course, you have to watch for your bidders and sell to the amount they're bidding. You guys could go home and practice and you'll be amazed how much fun it is, and how up-to-speed you are, after a little work."

The sale was about to resume. The boys hadn't brought a lunch, but they weren't thinking of food. The crowd moved towards the truck's new location. The churn went up on the table, and from that time on, Hal and Bobby pitched in, holding up items and watching for bids. They didn't ask if they could help out, they just did, lifting items and holding them up for the crowd to see. The Higgins brothers encouraged them, referring to them as "auction assistants".

Riley stuck around till the sale was nearly over. "You guys need a ride home?" Reluctantly, they waved to the auctioneers, signaling their departure.

John took a moment and said, "Ladies and gentlemen, let's hear it for our volunteer auction assistants."

Hal and Bobby waved as the crowd offered their applause, and before getting back to selling, Ron said, "I predict - future auctioneers!"

Bobby owed Riley eight dollars and promised to pay right away. They hauled their loot to the truck and Riley pulled into Fiske's yard first, so they could unload their treasures. Bessie and Stanley were thrilled with the gifts the boys had bid on and won for Fred and Colleen. Stanley quickly paid Bobby's debt and gave Hal the amount of cash he had spent on the dishes. Bessie filled the dishpan with warm water to give everything a thorough cleaning.

Bobby and Hal rushed off to the woodshop, eager to start practicing. First, they went at the numbers, at the same time, each on a different roll. Bobby was counting by tens' and Hal tried out 2.50, 5, 7.50, 10, 12.50, 15. They could hardly wait to throw in some filler words. Ron was right. They were better than they thought, and they could speak faster than they imagined was possible.

They would for sure be watching for the next Higgins auction. Usually, sales were held on the weekend. John told them they were welcome to help out any time.

"Next time we'll pay a little for your trouble." The boys were ecstatic. This day could not have been any better! For Bobby, the auction eased the sting of Fred's leaving. This was something different and something he just might be able to do. Ron seemed to think so, anyway.

As soon as Hal got home, he told his mother, and Dorie who was home for the weekend, that he had spent the day at Olsen's farm auction. He caught them by surprise as he suddenly crossed the room and held his mother's hand in the air, "How much am I bid for this grumpy, old chicken woman? I'm bid at one now, I'm bid at two now, will ya give me three?"

Dorie burst out laughing. "Stop it, Hal, you can't sell off your mother!"

Hal continued in his newfound, sing-song auctioneer voice.

"Okay, can't sell the old lady. How about the chickens? We have 78 chickens to sell today and every one of them full of lice. I'm bid one hundred dollars now, I'm bid two hundred dollars now, I'm bid three hundred dollars now. SOLD to the chicken woman herself! Three hundred bucks!"

Thea laughed till her shoulders shook. Hal was the only one who could make her laugh.

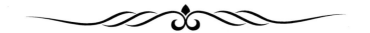

FARM WEDDING

The Big Clock struck eleven bells in June to mark Maggie Andersen's eleventh birthday. Back then, she had counted on Dorie coming home for the summer, but that plan got canceled because of Muriel. Stanley and Bessie promised to take her to the fair, but that wasn't till August. So, the main and only event coming up was Fred's wedding in July.

When school was over for the summer, Maggie was at the neighbors' house every day, helping Bessie with the yard since the wedding would be held outside. Bobby and Hal, with some direction from Stanley, built and painted an archway, crisscrossing laths to make a lattice effect for the bride and groom to stand in front of for the 'I do's'. Maggie added flowers from the garden and green poplar leaves, cut that morning. The arch was simple but impressive, creating an attractive backdrop for the pictures.

The special day dawned bright and clear, perfect for the outdoor wedding. The ceremony was set for 6 o'clock, followed by supper served on long tables near the garden. They arranged to have it late in the day so the farmers could do a day's work before it started, and the ladies who were doing the food would have lots of time to do the last-minute preparation.

Stanley was the one who had suggested the time. "There are no rules about the time of a wedding. We can do it at midnight if we want to!"

Considerable attention had been paid to wearing apparel for the occasion. Thea's green and white dress bought the year before, hung in the closet, as it had since the day of the doctor's appointment when she had angered Stanley. She did receive an invitation, but her pride kept her at home across the road, rather than going over to con-

53

gratulate young Fred, who had done so many caring acts of kindness for her since she moved there.

Maggie donned the yellow dress, also bought from the catalog the previous summer. It was quite short on her now, as she had sprouted like a wild weed in the past months. Her dress was set off with the now too tight, pointy-toed, boots, and she was a curious sight to behold as she and Dorie took a quick walk to the wedding next door.

Bessie often described her family as "down-home folks, and not a bit fussy." They struggled with what to wear to the wedding. Fred and Stanley were in line for proper suits and they each bought a dark-colored one they could tolerate, after a painful shopping trip to Stillwater. Bessie fared more comfortably the same day, as she and her friend Lil were dropped off at Fanny's Ladies Wear. She chose a loose fitting rose-colored dress, with pintucks across the front. A black half-hat with a net and a rose fabric flower capped off a mother-of-the-groom look.

Bobby agreed to wear new, pleated pants and a blue shirt, but he insisted there would be no monkey suit for him! When Hal saw the pants, he groaned with envy, wishing for some just like them.

"I got a job, Bobby, just last night. With my first paycheck, I'm getting me some duds like that!" His job was loading and unloading freight at the railway tracks. According to Hal, the boss was an old geezer who sat in a shack by the track counting the workers' hours.

"Sounds like heavy work," Bobby commented.

Ever the optimist, Hal replied, "I'll toughen up. The money sounds good to me!" The idea of cash appealed to Bobby, too, but with Fred moving out, Stanley would need help on the farm, and there were no wages for working at home.

The wedding guests were milling around the yard, visiting and watching for the bride's arrival. Right on time, at 5 minutes to 6, a late model car pulled into the driveway and parked by the house. The beaming bride emerged from the back seat, straightening and smoothing her poufy, white wedding dress. Fred was beside her in a second, elated that their day had come at last. Colleen's uncle had the honor of chauffeuring the bride, and several of the guests gathered around to look over the blue and white Chevy as he parked it in the shade.

Colleen's parents did not appear to be nostalgic or reluctant; perhaps they were even somewhat eager to hand over their daughter to this ambitious, hardworking, young farmer. Her father, Paul Krydor, took off his suit jacket as soon as he arrived, and left it in his brother's car until it was time to take a photo of the wedding couple with their parents. He well may have felt as uneasy in a suit as Stanley and Fred did. Colleen's mother, Mary Ann, was in her glory. She wore a fitted, kelly green suit with a belt. No doubt a tight girdle was the key to her flat stomach. She had a loud voice and was not shy. She ordered her younger daughter, Pauline, to get her a glass of lemonade almost as soon as they got out of the vehicle.

There were no other children in attendance and Bessie was quick to introduce Colleen's young sister to Maggie. The girl quickly reported back to her mother. "That girl can't talk! She won't say a word!"

"I know that Pauline. She's a mute. Colleen told us all about her. It's called a mute."

Her loud explanation drew unwanted attention, but Pauline was a confident sort and took over the situation. She was not at all short of words and as Maggie came up with nods and gestures, the girls spent the rest of the day together. They sneaked food before it was time to eat and made plans to become pen pals. Maggie didn't know much about writing a letter, not a real one that would go in the post office, but she was certain Bessie would help to keep in touch with her new friend.

Pauline had short, blond hair and wore a red plaid dress. Maggie didn't think much of the dress but she liked the girl's white sandals. Maggie slipped off her tight-fitting boots when it started to get dark, as they were hurting her feet something fierce. She knew if anyone noticed, they wouldn't care. She was just the neighbor kid from across the road, not a family member.

Dorie looked thoughtful as the vows were repeated after the minister: *for better, for worse, for richer, for poorer, in sickness and in health.* There was a day when Dorie had an intense crush on their neighbor Fred, but as she got older and lived in town, she figured she could do better. Fred's heart was stuck on farming and she had her sights set on what she thought of as "the high life". She had plans for herself, and those plans definitely did not include becoming a stodgy farm wife, or taking a job in piddly Stillwater. She expected to move to a bustling city, like Winnipeg or Vancouver. Every young girl has fanciful dreams, and as Dorie sat on a hard bench at Fred Fiske's wedding, wearing a pretty blue dress and listening to the bride say "I do", she reaffirmed her determination. She was sure she could do better than Fred, way better!

Dorie slipped away from the festivities shortly after the ceremony. Bessie spoke so kindly to her that she felt a twinge of guilt for her former thoughts about farmers' wives. As she was about to leave, Stanley was there to say goodbye. Before she knew it, her eyes filled with tears and she blurted out something she had not planned to say.

"Thank you, Stanley, for being so good to my little sister."

He nodded, acknowledging her appreciation. Always there was kindness in his eyes, especially towards the Andersen's.

"Take care of yourself, Dorie. We miss you around here."

The Fiskes had "done themselves proud." The food was bountiful and delicious - farm cooking at its finest, and served by several ladies from the community. Bessie's friend, Lil, reminded her a couple of times when she saw Bessie anxiously checking over the tables, "You are the mother-of-the-groom today, and you need to trust the work to us."

The evening flew by, and soon the smiling couple left the party, blowing the horn as they disappeared out the lane. A long string of tin cans bounced along behind the truck. Hal had enlisted Maggie and Pauline to secretly help him with that task as Bobby was not interested. The truck coughed a little as it rounded the corner heading north. The guests clapped and whistled. Bobby stood alone, leaning against the woodshop, watching them go. The honeymoon house at McKeen awaited Fred and his bride.

Pauline and Maggie's budding friendship was off to a promising start. They said goodbye a few times on the way to the uncle's car.

Pauline called out several farewell remarks.

"Don't forget to write."

"See you soon!"

"Goodbye, goodbye!"

Maggie waved furiously in response and was still pumping her arm when the Krydors left the yard.

Those who came by horse and buggy had set out for home before dusk. There was an empty feeling in the air as the final guests dispersed. Fred was gone. Maggie could tell Stanley, Bessie and Bobby were feeling it, too.

"I wonder if Colleen is a boss-cat," Maggie thought, fondly remembering the times Fred had rescued her from ridicule and being called "Maggie Rooster".

When the last car disappeared, Hal told Maggie it was time to go. Bessie had tears in her eyes, no doubt crying over Fred growing up. She hugged Maggie and said, "You were a big help getting the yard ready, Maggie. I'm glad *you're* not going anywhere just yet!"

Darkness had settled in. Maggie was still scared of the dark, as she had been as a little girl begging to sleep in Dorie's room, and so she was happy to walk with her brother.

As soon as they got on the path towards home, Hal remarked, "I wanted to stay and hang out with Bobby, but he's in a sour mood. I'll just leave him alone for now."

Maggie was frustrated with Hal's lack of compassion. She said nothing aloud of course, but her thoughts were very loud. "Don't you see he's sad? Can't you feel his sadness?"

When they got to the yard, a pack of coyotes started up a frenzied, yapping chorus, punctuated by high-pitched howls. They were a little too close for comfort. No doubt the smell of Maw's chickens was an overwhelming temptation. In the shadows, they could see a form standing beside the henhouse wall. They had a feeling it was Thea out there, standing on guard for her precious flock.

Maggie poked Hal on the shoulder. She was asking, in her silent way, "What's she got?"

Hal whispered in his sister's ear, "She's riding herd with her gun on those foul fowls of hers!" Maggie covered her mouth with her hand, shaking with laughter. What she would have replied, if she could have, was this: "What the heck is she doing with that gun? She couldn't hit the barn door with it, let alone a coyote!"

LOST AT SEA

They were like ships lost at sea - a 15-year-old farm boy who worried over everything, especially going to town school in the fall, and a harum-scarum girl of 11, who noiselessly wandered here and there, always alone and always silent. Of course, the two of them were stuck on the wide-open prairie, but all the same, to say they were "lost ships" was an apt description. Like untethered vessels on rough water, they were insecure and disconnected from their surroundings, as they bobbed on the heaving water throughout that long and uncertain summer of 1944.

Hal came up with the bright idea of memorizing the Morse code, as well as the sound signals for boat safety on the water. It seemed pointless to Maggie for them to learn anything about boats, as they didn't even get to a lake. Still, Hal persisted, as he was smart and always eager to try out something new.

He studied the language of sound signals from a book he had taken from the school. One prolonged blast is the warning for danger. Two short blasts mean, "I intend to pass you on the starboard side." Three short blasts warn, "I'm backing up!"

Maggie thought about different signals, the kind that people give out, even when they don't make a sound. She was sure Bobby was giving off signs. He withdrew from the family. That had to mean something. Maggie knew enough to skedaddle when his signals indicated she wasn't welcome in the woodshop. Bobby and Hal practiced the boat signals. The SOS was particularly annoying - three dots, three dashes, and three dots. S-O-S!

If Bobby was giving off personal warning signals, they were lost in the heat of the afternoons and carried away on the hot, dry wind.

His thoughts were dark during haying, and as the infernal cows kept getting out, fencing had become a daily priority.

Bobby and his brother Fred had no opportunity to interact when the family met at the river. Fred was eager to talk to his dad about the rented farm and what all needed to be fixed on the house there. Of course, it was Fred's first go at farming on his own, and Stanley was always available for help and advice as he had promised on the wedding day. The river was a pleasant spot for a picnic, and even though Stanley's truck coughed and sputtered most of the way, they made it to their designated meeting place. Hal had invited himself to come along.

Fred seemed to get a kick out of Hal. The guy was funny, and thrived on getting laughs wherever he went. Hal was in fine form that Sunday afternoon, cracking jokes.

He got their attention by asking, "Did you hear about the time Fred Fiske left home and wasted all his money? He wrote a postcard home. 'No mon, no fun, your son' and Stanley Fiske wrote back, 'Too bad, so sad, your dad'!" Fred and his parents hooted at his joke. The more Fred appeared to enjoy Hal's entertainment, the more invisible Bobby felt. Just before they all parted company, to head for home and milking cows, Bobby tuned into his dad's conversation with Fred.

"I was going to send Bobby home with you today to help with your fencing, but now the hay is ready."

Bobby hadn't heard about going to Fred's. That would have been swell, the best thing possible in this stinking summer. He heard Fred's answer loud and clear and felt the sting of his words.

"Oh, that's okay, Dad. Bobby's a hard worker, but I know you need him. I think I can hire one of the neighbor boys instead. Their dad is a tough boss and they say all his kids know how to earn a day's pay.

Bobby remembered that conversation as the following week unfolded in the heat of the hayfield. No problem! Fred could easily hire someone else. It didn't seem to matter to Fred if it was his brother or a stranger. Bobby's thoughts also strayed, as they did so often, to school starting in the fall. Only one month away.

On a Saturday morning, Stanley and his son went into town to pick up the cream check and buy groceries. Bessie usually went along to do her shopping, but for the past week she had been feeling poorly. She said her diabetes was acting up.

Stanley parked the truck between the post office and the railway station and started down the board sidewalk for the mail. Bobby jumped out of the truck to retrieve the empty cream can off the green wooden wagon at the train station. "S. Fiske" was hand-painted on the side of the cream can. It was the one right on the edge. Bobby swung it down from the wagon. As he turned to go back to the truck, a face appeared beside the station door, and a voice hissed at him, easily heard by anyone and everyone who happened to be nearby.

"Hey, Kisser!" The cream can rolled in the dust. Two strides and Oliver was in the air. When he came down, he landed on his back and felt heavy farm boots pounding his ribs.

Bobby was way out of control. "I'll kill you, so help me, I will kill you." Stanley was suddenly on one side of Bobby and the drayman on the other, pulling him back.

"He's not worth your time, Son," Stanley said, dragging Bobby towards the truck. They left Oliver writhing on the ground like the snake he was.

Stanley loaded the cream can and they headed for home, not bothering to go to the store.

Stanley was exasperated. "Why didn't you let me handle it, Bobby?"

"Back off, Dad. From now on, I'll take care of myself." Stanley tried to talk it out when they got home, but Bobby's face was red and he was fuming. It was a silent rage. He had nothing to say to anyone. He no longer needed his big brother or his dad for protection. He had all the steam he needed to take care of himself. He stayed angry the rest of the day, and the rest of the week - and onward.

Stanley suggested a drive up to the north field to check the fence line. He tossed the keys to his son, but Bobby turned and walked out of the house, allowing the keys to land on the floor. He sought refuge in his woodshop.

Stanley and Bessie talked late into the night. "I can't believe how mad he is. It's not like him. He said he'd kill the kid."

"How long has this been building, do you think?"

"I don't know. It sneaked up on me."

Stanley arranged a meeting with Dr. Marshall. "My boy is angry."

"Often adolescent boys, even with mild facial differences, become withdrawn and are subject to aggression and depression. Are you seeing symptoms of that nature?"

Stanley rubbed his chin. "That's exactly why I'm here."

The doctor's words fit Bobby to a "T". Bobby now pulled away from everyone around him, and was constantly in a bad mood. His concerned parents witnessed what they had never seen before in their youngest son. He was beyond angry and he didn't hold back.

Fred Fiske was a one-of-a-kind brother, and while he attended the same school as Bobby, he was his protector. Even later, when Bobby went alone to the one-room school down the road, the students there were well aware that Fred was not far away. A big brother is gift from heaven, especially if you are self-conscious and have endured some bullying in the past.

But now Fred was married and had moved with the wife to McKeen. Town school was looming for Bobby, and he would be totally on his own, now that Hal wasn't coming. The distress signals may have been faint, but they were real.

The kicker to it all happened on the last Saturday morning in July. Bobby rode to town with his dad to get staples, those curved, sharp-on-both-end nails necessary for fastening barbed wire to the fence posts. Stanley always called them "steeples" but Bobby had taken note of the sign on the barrel they came out of the last time they were there. They were rightly called staples. Stanley prided himself in keeping his fence line perfectly straight and the three strands of wire a uniform distance apart.

They rattled into town and pulled up in front of the hardware store. Once inside, Stanley went through the side door to the lean-to looking for George Marshall. He was there, and so were the wooden boxes and nail kegs holding various bolts, washers, different kinds of nails, and screws.

"Need some steeples."

"What do you need, a couple of pounds?"

"Yeah, that should do it."

Meanwhile out in the main part of the store, Bobby waited near the counter, looking at the display of small items. At the far end of the long counter, sitting on a nail keg, was Cecil Grange. Bobby had seen him before. Not a nice guy. His stringy hair stuck out the back of a greasy black cap. A line of chewing tobacco juice ran down one side of his mouth. He stared at Bobby as if sizing him up.

After a minute or two, he said loudly, "Whoa there, Boy, you better put that back!"

Bobby looked around to see who he was talking to. Cecil's weasely face and beady eyes were honed in on him. His cynical smile showed his tobacco-stained teeth.

"In this here store, we pay for what we take home."

Bobby snapped back, "I don't know what you're talking about."

"Oh, I think you do. There were half a dozen screwdrivers right there beside you a minute ago. I see only three now. Better cough up!"

Fred Fiske was known to have blown his top and been in a serious scrap or two in the past, but Bobby had the reputation of "the quiet one". Not this summer.

On his way to Cecil's perch, Bobby growled, "We'll see who'll cough up! You're lying and you know it. I didn't take anything."

Still determined to push it, Cecil squeaked, "And I say you did."

The commotion brought Stanley and George out of the lean-to. Stanley carried a large brown paper package, tied with string and already paid for. Bobby and the older man were having a stand-off. Bobby's face was almost purple.

Cecil spoke up quickly. "Sorry to tell you, George, but this customer here is a little light-fingered. He just swiped three of your screwdrivers off the counter there."

Stanley stepped between them. Six inches from the weasel's face he roared, "You're a liar!"

"I swear I saw him do it and he's laughing about it, too." Bobby's surgery had left him with a somewhat upturned lip on the right side. The guy was making fun of him for sure. Stanley had big mitts. His strong fingers locked onto Cecil's neck muscle As they approached the door, Cecil whined, "I was just funnin', just funnin'!"

The powerful shove at the door sent him stumbling outside, raising up dust as he barely managed to keep his balance. George stood beside Stanley, a look of pure disgust on his face.

"He's a no-good!" He looked at Bobby's still beet-red face, and said, "Pay him no mind, Son. He's the scum of the earth! You won't find him in here again."

The Fiske men wasted no time getting into the truck. Bobby said nothing all the way home. The humiliation was enough to silence him, and besides, he had nothing to add to his father's choice words.

When they got out of the truck, the heat was staggering. Bobby said, "I'm done, Dad. Can we do it tomorrow?"

"Tomorrow's Sunday."

Stanley attempted to place his hand on his son's shoulder. "Bobby…"

But the boy had already turned away, heading to his refuge, the little woodshop in the shade of the trees. Stanley loaded the truck with the post hole auger, some posts, the bag of staples, and the hammer. Bessie came out with a two quart sealer of cold water. The truck moved on down the fence line to where the cows had broken through again. Bobby would come later.

TRASHING THE WOODSHOP

Sometimes Maggie sent out her own distress signals, like the day she trashed Bobby's woodshop. Her signals were muffled, as she did not speak in front of anyone except Bessie and Stanley, and her words to them were rare now. They were privileged to have gained her trust, but it seemed they were losing her. So for her benefit and theirs, they continued to hire her for yard work.

The timing was poor. While Bobbly was having a set-to with Cecil Grange in town, Maggie had been busy creating havoc in his hide-out. He easily caught her as she flew barefoot down the shortcut path towards her yard. Usually, she evaded consequences to her behavior, but he grabbed her skinny arm, and she knew there was no escape. He hauled her back across the plowed field between their two houses and shoved her through the open door of his beloved woodshop. She had done a job of it all right!

Bobby crossed his arms and blocked the doorway.

"Clean it up!" This was the angriest she had ever seen him. Just how angry he was, she didn't want to know. She felt an unfamiliar tinge of fear. Usually, nothing fazed her. She'd had enough switchings in her lifetime to know what was coming when Thea vented her fury, but this was new. Bobby had never laid a hand on her.

She was unsure of what he would do next, and knowing he was more irritable this summer than he had ever been, she saw no retreat. He glared at her as if she were a piece of dirt. He looked "fit to be tied".

The girl was fast, he had to admit that. With lightning speed she stacked the wood pieces back in their piles and lined up the tools in order, trying to remember exactly where they belonged. The shavings she had dumped out of a box by the door made the most mess, but she painstakingly swept them up. Bobby's whittling tools were damaged. The blades were bent, and one was broken right off. What she had done with them, Bobby couldn't imagine, but here she was standing in front of him with the sorry-looking knives on her outstretched palm.

"Why do you want to be like your mother?"

Maggie quickly shrugged her thin shoulders, and then the full impact of his words hit her. She vigorously shook her head, hair flying across one side of her face and then the other. She couldn't stop. With words locked inside, she had no better means of communication. When Bobby spoke, his voice was flat.

"Don't be like her, Maggie. She's mean, and you're better than this!"

They finished the tidying job together in silence. Bobby slipped the damaged whittling tools into a drawer. Maggie fiddled with a couple of pieces of wood, aimlessly trying to fit together some kind of creation.

There were diamond willow sticks behind the door, and Bobby selected two. On a previous Sunday when the family met Fred and Colleen at the river for a picnic, he and Hal had discovered a willow bush with the diamond-shaped indentations. Bobby got a hack saw from the back of the truck and they cut off several suitable lengths for walking sticks. He intended to strip the bark, and smooth and sand the surfaces until the natural colors showed through.

He handed the smaller one to Maggie and took another for himself. They sat together on the bench outside the woodshop door, paring off long strips of brown bark.

Maggie wouldn't, or couldn't, bring herself to show her repentance. That was foreign to her. The fact she sat with him carefully stripping off bark, and not running away was enough to show him she was not likely to do it again. He assumed they had arrived at that understanding. Maggie's stick was the perfect height for her. That is, if she ever finished it and slowed down long enough to make use of it.

Bessie had observed the woodshop incident - first from the kitchen window, as she witnessed the commotion when Maggie was brought back to the yard. Bobby, usually passive, showed dark anger on his flaming face, as he had roughly steered Maggie along the path. Bessie wasted no time. She ambled out to the garden that just happened to be next to Bobby's woodshop, and there she held vigil. She heard the whole thing and saw some of it.

When the diamond willow walking sticks had been put away for further work another day, and Maggie had taken off once again, Bessie knocked on the half-closed door. No answer. She peeked around the door and saw Bobby stretched out on his make-shift bed. It was just a cot with an old blanket and pillow, something he had fixed up for hot summer nights. His eyes were closed.

"I was in the garden the whole time."

A slight nod from Bobby encouraged her to continue.

"You handled that well, Bobby, and I doubt she'll do it again. I just realized how lonely she is. She is certainly looking for attention."

"Well, she got it all right."

"Rightly so. Don't worry. She needed to know you were mad. You were firm and you were kind at the end."

Bobby had no reply. He looked exhausted, his face still flushed.

"Are you sleeping well, son?"

"Not really. I've got things on my mind."

"Well, it could be the heat," his mother remarked. "I noticed you didn't eat breakfast."

"Just not that hungry, Mom."

"Please don't be worrying over me, Bobby. The doctor and I have pretty well sorted out my diabetes issues. I'm trying to build up strength again. The problem is, I just don't have any oomph."

A couple of days later, Maggie gathered some daisies and snapdragons and asked if she could borrow a sealer. Bessie wondered if she might take them to her mother in a gesture of making peace.

Maggie poured water into the sealer and took it outside as the workday at Fiske's was over, and it was time to head home. Watchful as the hawk that constantly soared over Anderson's chicken coop, Bessie was at the window. She was not overly surprised when Maggie dropped off her peace offering at the door of Bobby's woodshop.

AT THE FAIR

The Ferris wheel could be seen for miles. Stanley wheeled his old truck through the gate, as the music from the midway carried across the fairgrounds. The men who collected the money for entrance tickets wore navy blue bib aprons, with separate compartments for bills and change. Visors were pulled low over their eyes to protect them from the sun. It was already hot, and they would have a long and busy day, judging by the vehicles already lined up to the highway.

The annual Stillwater Fair had been in operation for over 50 years, and even though it had to be toned down a lot in the '30s due to the depression, no money, and next-to-no farm produce to show, it still existed. This year, 1944, it promised to be a big one. No one would be disappointed.

Maggie rode in the middle of the front seat, between Bessie and Stanley. It was a secure feeling for her and it was easy to imagine she was their kid. Hal and Bobby felt the excitement, as they stood up from the egg crates they had been sitting on in the truck box.

There was a lot to see - the barns, the long white exhibition tents near the road, and a huge parking area where some horses, buggies, and wagons were lined up, not far from the rows of vehicles. Numerous Indian tents were set up on the south side of the entrance, and the boys could smell smoke from their small fires. They could see the grandstand where the evening performance would take place. From those high bleachers, pretty well everyone would get a bird's-eye view of the show at the end of the day.

Music blared from loudspeakers that were fastened on poles and buildings. The midway boasted a myriad of rides, and each played its own music. Their flashing lights would show up when the sun went down. Screams from the riders on the spinning tilt-a-whirl set Hal's blood racing. He could hardly wait to try it out, and to explore the rows of dark-colored tents.

Stanley parked the truck not far from the action. They heard the barkers over a loudspeaker, repeating, "Three for a buck, try your luck." Balloons and darts were set up, and the prizes were displayed high and out of reach. They were large, colorful ornaments that appeared to be made of plaster of paris.

"See Tom Thumb, the smallest man on earth. Only a dime! Come on in to the house of mirrors! More fun than a barrel of monkeys!" Their words sparked curiosity, adding mystery and wonder to this day at the fair.

Before they left home home, Stanley told the boys to keep their money buttoned up in their front shirt pockets and to keep an eye out for crooks. He explained to them the danger of pickpockets. Maggie had never heard the word "pickpocket" before, but by the end of Stanley's warning she was relieved she had given Bessie her bit of spending money for safe keeping.

"It's not the local people we're talking about," Bessie added. "When the fair comes to town, a lot of strangers show up from who knows where. We're not saying they're bad people, just reminding you to be careful."

Bessie had worked on her fair entries for the past two months. The Agricultural Society kept the farm women's interest high by mailing out specifications for the exhibits. There were prizes to be won for sewing items, knitting, needlework, rugs, quilts, and baked goods. When Bessie first encouraged Maggie to enter some handcrafts, she was met with a shrug and zero interest; however, the girl pricked up her ears as she took note of the different categories. Maggie eagerly picked chokecherries and saskatoons from the bushes in the pasture, as well as raspberries and strawberries from the garden. Bessie went to work making jams and jellies. The exhibition was always held in August when farm produce was at its best.

Maggie selected and washed garden vegetables, and grouped them according to the regulations: three carrots, one cabbage, five pounds of potatoes. She cut flowers early in the morning so they would be fresh. One category was for a wildflower arrangement and the other was a bouquet of garden flowers.

Bessie looked forward to adding all their items to the display tables, with help from Stanley and Maggie. Her apple pie looked about perfect as she padded it carefully with plenty of newspapers for transport to the fair. Perhaps by the time they located the boys for lunch, she could proudly add the prizewinning apple pie to the menu. Maggie also looked forward to their picnic together. She noticed some families had spread blankets on the ground and were sitting in the shade.

There was a large tent with a sign, "School Exhibits". Maggie wondered if Miss Newberry had entered any of her students' work. She hadn't mentioned it, so probably not.

Hal and Bobby headed straight for the midway while Stanley, Bessie, and Maggie carried load after load to the long display tables. Maggie fluffed up her flower bouquets and Stanley helped place them in the correct spot. For such a young girl, she had a flair for design and arrangements. Could she win? It didn't matter if she did or not. This was the highlight of the summer for her. It was a day at the fair, far from Thea and a hot day in the Andersen yard.

Maggie spied a pony ring as they carried items into the exhibition tent. She had never tried to ride their horse, the one Hal called Old Nag, but now she wondered as she looked closely at the ponies, what it would be like to take a horse ride. She felt a little sorry for the ponies as they circled round and round, but the children riding looked as if their faces would split with delight.

"I think I'd like a pony of my own." Of course, she didn't say it aloud. It was a thought that jumped into her head. She imagined owning the middle-sized one there, the brown one with a black mane and tail and a red bridle. Imagine galloping around the countryside or to school on a pony. He could be her best friend. There would be nothing wrong with having a pony for a friend.

A pig catching contest was scheduled for 2 o'clock, and Hal was crazy about the idea. The prize was a dollar and he figured on winning. He outran all the students at Aroma School, and won first again, when three other schools competed at the field day. Hal planned exactly how he would grab the pig's hind leg with both hands and hang on, even if it dragged him.

"Come on, Bobby, let's both enter!" Bobby shook his head.

Stanley promised Maggie he would take her on the Ferris wheel in the evening so they could look down at the fairgrounds and see the lights of the city from the top. Throughout the afternoon, she was content to stay with Bessie at the exhibits. She wished she had entered additional categories like bundles of wheat, oats and barley. Maybe next year.

Hal and Bobby heard the food vendors yelling, "Peanuts! Popcorn!" The air was heavy with the smell of onions and hot cooking oil. The exciting atmosphere had gripped them both, especially Hal, as he discreetly extracted a dime from his meager stash of coins and exchanged it for a swirl of pink cotton candy.

Most of the tents along the way were closed up to hide whatever was inside, so it must have been hot as blazes in there. There were signs on each tent and the first one they saw was printed in large red letters. FREAK SHOW. Outside, two men took turns shouting to the passersby, "Ten cents for a peek in each booth! Come inside and you'll get an eyeful! Ruby, the bearded woman, Go-go our five-legged dog! Step right up."

He looked directly at Hal. "Hey, good lookin'. Put down your money right here. You'll meet Lulu, the dancing lady who wears only two little hummingbird feathers that she plucked herself!"

Even Hal was horrified at that description. Lulu herself appeared on stage, wearing a scanty outfit in pink and black lace, crossing her high heels, one in front of the other. She looked fairly old with a fake smile and lots of lipstick. Hal and Bobby pushed through the crowd and when they were well away, Hal said, "Well, I would have liked to see the dog, maybe."

Bobby looked dour. "You don't need to pay to see a freak, Hal. You can see one any day of the week." The idea of paying to see people who were different, unnerved him. The lights came on for Hal. He realized then that Bobby was referring to himself as a freak. Bobby didn't look any different than other people but he *thought* he did. That was the sad part.

They moved on down the line to explore the games. This was more like it! People were laughing and having fun, spending a little here and there on a game of skill, hoping to win a prize. Hal and Bobby watched as some tried their luck spinning the Money Wheel, tossing dimes into a bottle, and throwing darts. It didn't take long for Hal to get in on the action.

Stanley went searching for Hal and Bobby. It would be a miracle to find them in this crowd. It didn't take very long, however, as the boys were already coming his way, both looking very distraught, but relieved when they caught a glimpse of his old felt hat.

"What's up?" Stanley asked. He had planned this outing carefully, hoping Bobbly would find some fun in it. So far, the summer had been a disaster for Bobby, which was mainly why Hal had been invited to come along to the fair. But Hal, the usually happy-go-lucky Hal, was looking at his boots.

It didn't take long for the story to come out. Hal had tried his luck first at the balloon and dart game and didn't win a thing, despite all the promises of the smooth-talking operator. The boys moved on to a shooting game with a small gun to aim at wooden yellow ducks, moving along a straight wire.

"All you gotta do is knock one down!"

Hal took aim and poof! One yellow duck bit the dust. He held out his hand for his prize, but the hawker said quickly, "Not so fast, you have to get three in a row!" Hal shot again. This time he missed, and a third shot went wide.

He turned the gun over in his hands, inspecting it. "Something's wrong with this gun."

The man gave Hal a condescending look. "The gun works fine. I'd say something's wrong with the shooter."

Hal was mad. He had already wasted 75 cents for nothing. The smooth talker kept Hal on the string. "Let's make a deal. The next shot is free. If you get it, and one other, I'll give you ten bucks." Ten bucks! Hal's greed got the better of him. He nearly nailed the next smiling yellow duck, but not quite.

Bobby yanked on Hal's shirt sleeve. "Come on, Hal, this is nuts. Get out while you can." But Hal was bit by the lure of gold, and it overpowered him. He turned away from the owner of the flock of ducks, and from his buttoned pocket, opened the envelope that held his wages from old Chrome-dome. It was his first pay, a whole month's worth of hard work, loading and unloading heavy freight at the rail yard. He turned back to face his challenge. This time he would show them all. They'd see there was nothing at all wrong with his shooting!

The ducks were going faster now, sailing swiftly along on the wire. Hal recklessly laid down a dollar and took a shot. Missed. Another. Missed. Another.

The smooth talker said, "I'll give you that one free, as a bonus. You're doing fantastic! Take another set!"

Hal laid down another dollar. Bobby walked away in disgust. Could Hal be that stupid? Anyone could see the thing was rigged. The yellow ducks were going so fast now, they were a blur. The wire must have been hooked to a motor under the pretend water beneath them. A crowd gathered around and cheered Hal on. If there ever was something Hal couldn't resist it was praise and attention.

By the time Bobby made his way back, Hal's face was red and he was sweating. He replaced the gun in its holder for the next stooge. They turned away, not looking at the crook who had talked Hal out of his wages.

Bobby asked quietly, "How much did he get?"

Hal didn't look up. His voice was barely audible. "He got it all."

Bobby and Hal headed back towards the exhibition tents and the parking area. They were looking for Stanley as they walked in the direction of the truck.

Stanley listened to Hal's tale of woe. Anyone watching would have seen the color rising on Stanley Fiske's neck. By the time they retraced their steps to the duck booth, Stanley's face was as fiery as Bobby had ever seen it.

The mouthy operator coaxed a girl and her boyfriend to each take a free shot. "Everybody plays, everybody wins!"

Stanley picked up speed as the boys pointed out the man who had swindled Hal out of his money. When Stanley's beet-red face was less than a foot away from the other man's chin, he said loudly, "Give this kid back his money!"

His words were met with a sneer. The swindler had run up against this situation many times before and was not about to lose what he had already taken.

"The kid can't shoot. Anybody else could have at least broke even. He lost out, fair and square."

"There is no fair and square here," Stanley said evenly. "You're as crooked as they come, and I'll make sure all your other customers know it!" He placed his hands on either side of the man and gripped the little doorway to the back of the tent. The guy was pinned.

The man looked from side to side at the dispersing crowd, and at Bobby and Hal. "Hand over his money."

Another sneer. "Are you his daddy?"

"You bet I'm his daddy!"

The duck man's clothes were dirty. He shoved his grimy hand into his pants' pocket, and pulled out a wad of bills.

"Take it and go," he snarled. Stanley knew when he was ahead. Grabbing each boy by the forearm, he hustled them down the dusty track towards the parking area. Stanley poured water into the enamel cups Bessie had packed with the noon lunch. The boys each took a long, slow drink. Hal sheepishly looked at Stanley, whose face had by now returned to its natural color.

Stanley handed the wad of money to Hal. There was no "I hope you've learned your lesson." All he said was, "I hope you didn't lose too much of it, Son."

"Thanks, Daddy," was all Hal could muster.

Bessie and Maggie had won some ribbons already. All five of them took a walk through the barns. Maggie saw the biggest pig she had ever seen. It was white and huge. A gigantic team of Percheron horses wore frilly red and gold ribbons clipped to their bridles. Goats and sheep, were on display in the clean stalls. A magnificent Hereford bull caught the attention of everyone touring the barns. There were many fine specimens from different farms, all vying for a ribbon and a few bucks for first, second and third prize.

Hal looked for the pig he would be chasing. For now, the exhilarating fun had gone out of the day, but he still wanted to make a dive for that hog. The gambler in him was confident he just might win!

The day progressed as they took in the exciting sights and sounds of a day at the fair. Maggie eyed up the merry-go-round. They nearly passed it by, but as Stanley saw there was no line-up, he offered to buy her a ticket.

"How about a horse ride just before the Ferris wheel, Maggie?"

Maggie tried to look disinterested, giving the impression she was too old for it. Hal caught on and said quickly, "Come on, Sis, I've got some extra tickets." The others stared at Hal in surprise. Did he have any money left at all? He'd been on the rides all afternoon. No doubt all the money Stanley had recovered had been spent ten different ways by now!

Hal pulled a couple of crumped tickets out of his jeans pocket. Before Maggie knew it, her brother had pushed her in front of him, up onto the circular platform.

"Pick your ride," the operator called, "and make it quick!" Maggie could see the horses were painted different colors. The first one she saw was white and black with a silver saddle. She almost climbed up on it but then, she spied a brown pony with a black mane and tail - and wouldn't you know it - there was a red bridle and reins. It was just like the live one she had seen at the pony ring earlier in the day. In two seconds, she was in place, holding on to the pole that her horse was attached to. Hal was right beside her on a sparkling, all-gold horse.

The ride began to move. Slowly at first, the horses went up and down to the music. First, Maggie's steed was high at the top of the pole. Next, it was Hal's. Maggie was grinning just like the kids at the pony ring, but she couldn't help it. The music, oh the music, of a merry-go-round! She had heard nothing like it before. As the ride revolved, they approached the family waiting on the sidelines. Maggie could see Bessie nodding in time to the music, no doubt humming along. When she asked her later, Bessie said it was an old waltz her mother loved and was called, "Over the Waves". The organ played the song at a fast clip to match the speed of the horses.

Ever the clown, Hal waited till they had circled directly beside the others, and pretended to be a cowboy. He waved his hat at them and yelled, "Yahoo!" Bobby turned away in embarrassment but Stanley waved, and Bessie yelled as they went past, "Ride 'em, Cowboy!" The ride sped up - up and down, around and around. Maggie couldn't wipe the grin off her face!

On the way to the grandstand, they all stopped at the Ferris wheel. With fear and trembling, Maggie stepped up on the ride with Stanley and wiggled into the swinging seat. A safety bar was locked in front of them and she hung on for dear life. They were going high. It wouldn't take much for a skinny girl to go skidding off the seat and out into the wild, blue yonder.

Bessie had reassured her. "You'll be fine. Just take a look at the lights for me."

Hal and Bobby clambered onto the next seat. The Ferris wheel was a one-ticket ride. The wilder rides required two. Suddenly, they were moving! Splendid music began to play, and the swaying seat climbed up and up. Maggie held on, frozen with fear and delight.

When they reached the top, Stanley looked out at the country-side, beyond the city. "Now would you look at that! I can nearly see our farm from up here." It was the truth. They could see for miles. At that moment Maggie felt free as a bird. This was something she had dreamed of doing, but she didn't know it would be like this. Around and around they went. The song changed to a different one, a sad song, as they gazed down at the lights of the city. She thought of the Big Clock's pendulum, swinging back and forth in time to the beat of the music.

The grandstand was grand indeed, featuring a troupe of pol-ished performers who maneuvered an impressive high wire act. Their glittering costumes shimmered in the lights. The show ended with a smiling cowboy and his guitar, singing everyone back to their vehi-cles for the ride home.

Bessie held Maggie's hand as throngs of people moved towards the parking lot. About the time they found the truck, they heard a low, booming sound. Was it thunder? Suddenly, the sky was ablaze with bursts of color - purple, green, red, gold and silver - exploding in the sky to the east of the fairgrounds. Fireworks! It was a gala send-off!

The boys hunkered down in the back of the truck. They put on their jackets against the chilly wind. Hal was still buzzed by his day at the fair and began to sing at the top of his lungs. He had heard a song on the radio, "So Long, It's Been Good to Know You," and he made up his own nonsensical words to it. "So Long, Spitz a goal-yuh". He sang the same line over and over as the stars came out and the wind died down and the truck steadily pressed towards home. Hal had somehow missed his appointment with the pig, but he wasn't bothered by that.

Bobby marveled at his friend. When they both were sick and tired of the "spitza goal-yuh" song, Hal lit into a couple of other tunes. He was never worried about what others would think. Bobby understood they were made of different stuff. When Hal had something on his mind, he talked or yelled, or sang. When Bobby was troubled, he kept it all inside. After all that had happened since morning, especially Hal gambling away his paycheck and then depending on Stanley to get it back, Bobby wondered how Hal could shuck it off, and end the day in such a crazy mood.

Bobby thought of his day at the fair. He remembered the word "freaks" in large red letters, and the dirt and the grime in the air. He knew his parents had tried to set up a special day for him, but he really should have stayed at home.

AUCTION AUDITIONS

Riley announced there was to be an auction on the second Saturday in August at the old Holborn Hardware store. The building had been shut down for six months but finally, its contents were being disposed of. Riley heard the Higgins Brothers were billed to run the sale. Hal wasted no time running across the road to tell Bobby. While they were scheming how they could get there, Riley came by and offered a ride. They hadn't considered he would want to go, but Riley liked the atmosphere of an auction sale and he also was a bit of a junk collector. Bobby and Hal could hardly wait to see the Higgins men perform again, and they hoped they could help out.

The boys practiced in earnest before the sale, hoping to get an evaluation from their heroes. The auction was the only topic that could reach Bobby. With practice, the boys were getting better and faster. They could only wonder what John and Ron Higgins would think of their efforts.

Fred had left an old cowboy hat hanging on a nail in Fiske's barn. Colleen told Fred in no uncertain terms that she wasn't marrying a cowboy. She said she was marrying a farmer, and she wanted him to wear a felt hat as her father wore. So, the boys beat the dust out of Fred's castoff hat and then asked Bessie how to restore it. She cleaned it with a damp rag and then set about to steam and shape it using the kettle on the cook stove. That woman could work wonders! By the time she was done, the old hat for Hal looked way better than Bobby's newer one. So, Bessie gave it a working over, too.

On the day of the auction, the boys aspired to look like a couple of promising young auctioneers, as they approached the Higgins brothers. The older men registered surprise when they recognized

Bobby and Hal, and offered to hire them for the day. They were working alone, without an auction assistant, and the crowd was growing.

When they briefly took a break at noon, the men asked for a demonstration. Hal was only too eager. It was strange to Bobby how confident Hal was, especially since his mother had never given him any praise at home. How he pulled it out, Bobby would never know, but Hal put on a show and a half! He put everything he had into it. He was loud, he was sing-songy, and he had his filler words sliding in at the right time and place. The Higgins men sincerely commended him.

Ron said, "See, I told you, it's easier than you think. I can tell you've really been practicing. Good for you, Hal!"

The three of them turned their eyes expectantly to Bobby. Looking down, Bobby admitted, "I'm sorry, but I'm a self-conscious guy. I'll take a pass."

Hal, always eager to find a solution, put both hands on his friend's shoulders and turned him around, so his back was to the auctioneers.

"Okay, Bobby, do it this way. You don't have to look at them and they don't have to look at you. I'll be the bid catcher. Here, sell my hat."

Bobby had a lingering nasal sound when he spoke, due to his cleft lip and the resulting surgery. A unique sound came through loud and clear as Bobby launched into his auctioneer chant, do or die! He was easy to listen to and the numbers were clear. His sound was a cut above. He injected a little humor as he wound it up with, "Sold! Souvenir hat, worn by outlaw Hal Anderson at his hanging!"

The Higgins men nearly split a gut laughing. They had underestimated this lad's potential!

"You've got it, Bobby!"

Ron put his hand on Hal's arm. "Don't let this discourage you, Son. You're good. Keep working on it. But if I were to bet on who could make fame and fortune out of this, I'd put my money on this guy here." Bobby's face flushed red.

John nodded. "You've got something special there, Bobby. I wouldn't say it if it wasn't true."

The auctioneers were big talkers. John continued, "Let me give you a little history of American auctioneering. In England, they're very stiff with their polite and calculated selling. They speak like they're falling asleep, like this. 'Thank you, kind sir, for your bid of 9 pounds. Will anyone go 10?' Out here in North America, we have a different style. We do the auctioneer chant. Some people call it auctioneer fever. As you've observed, a big part of what we do is to keep the crowd revved up and bidding."

Ron chimed in. "The chant started after the Civil War in the States when they sold off mules and wagons and other war equipment to the Southerners, who desperately needed supplies. Only those military men who held the rank of "colonel" were allowed to do the selling. To this day, an excellent auctioneer is sometimes referred to as the "colonel". I have never personally had that compliment, but dang it, I'm making a prediction right now. If you ever decide to go into it as a business, Bobby, you'll have every right to use the name, 'Colonel Bob Auctions'."

The boys helped Riley put the boxes and junk he had bid on into the back of the truck. The three rode in the cab on the way home and Hal explained to Riley how the Higgins men had reacted to their auditions. Riley added his compliments when he heard about it. Easygoing Hal was content for his friend to get the glory.

"Well, from what they said, Pal, you'll be the big boss getting all the money. I'll be the sucker holding up sale items all day long till my arm falls off!"

MARK MY WORDS

Hal quit his job in town. When Stanley asked him what happened, he answered evasively, "Didn't work out." Stanley had tried to be a mentor to him as the boys were growing up, and so Hal was embarrassed to confess he was a quitter. When he first landed the job, he bragged about how much he was going to make working in town, and lorded it over Bobby.

Hal provided the details as he and Bobby headed out to the east field to shoot gophers. Both boys had been taught to safely handle a .22. Stanley had done well by his sons, and also Hal, in so many ways.

"Wasn't my fault, Bobby. The old Chrome-dome just sits around spying on the workers. Said we can't smoke on the job, but he leans back with a big, fat cigar, puffin' all day long, stinkin' up the whole place. He didn't like me from the start. He heard me call him an old geezer. I tried to tell him it was all in fun." Bobby raised his eyebrows, but didn't comment. Hal finished the story.

"So, he comes up to me and says, 'Well, big boy, you best be headin' home.' It wasn't even close to quitting time, so I told him I'd work till the end of the day. All of sudden he lost it, and fired his cane at me. I left, but he still owes me wages. I'm going to get them, too." Bobby didn't comment on Hal getting fired.

When the boys left the field, they went to the house for a drink. Maggie was there. She had picked two pails of peas from the garden and was sitting in the cool kitchen beside Bessie. The shared pail between them was for the discarded pea shells.

Hal had been gone for a couple of weeks working in town, and now that he was back, he seemed loud and pushy.

He looked at his sister and asked, "What's buzzin', cousin?" Hal was always trying out the new sayings he heard around town. Another new one was "hot diggity dog!" and he was watching for an opportunity to try it out.

Maggie liked her brother. He could usually make her laugh, and he talked enough for both of them. He had a certain way about him. He could liven up most situations, somewhat like Dorie's friend, Muriel had. Suddenly, Hal grabbed the pail of pea shells and held it in the air. He caught them all by surprise as he lit into his auctioneer chant, forming the words so fast, they could hardly believe it. He must have been practicing.

"Pea shells here. What am I bid? I'm bid one, I'm bid two. I'm bid three and four, where four? I'm bid four dollars! Sold!" He clapped his hands to finalize the sale. "Pea pods for the pigs!"

He handed the pail back to Bessie who was already laughing, as always, when anything tickled her. She said, "You're really good, Hal!"

"Oh, not as good as someone else we know. Did Bobby tell you what John and Ron Higgins said about us?"

Of course he hadn't. Bobby said very little to any of them the last while.

"Well, he gave us a few tips and after some practice, he wanted to hear us. I went first, and then Bobby took his turn. Higgins pointed right at this guy here, and said 'I'll give it to you straight. This is the one I would place my bet on. Bobby, you could make a living out of this. You've got the perfect voice for it'."

Bobby's parents looked surprised and pleased, and Bobby's face was flushed.

"C'mon Bobby, show your folks!"

Bobby shook his head. It was a definite no.

Hal was undaunted. Still determined to get something going, he looked at his sister and said, "Okay Maggie, today's the day. No actions or pointing, just answer my questions. How do you like your summer job with Bessie?"

Maggie looked trapped, glancing from side to side.

Hal urged her, "C'mon, Sis. You're not scared of these people. You're among friends."

Maggie opened her mouth and closed it. Stanley saw the panic in her eyes and her quick look at the door. He caught her hand before she could escape, and he didn't let go till he sat her down near Bessie again.

He said quietly, "It's okay, Love. Bessie and I understand."

He looked at Hal, and said kindly, "You can't force her. We've figured that out."

Maggie stared at the floor. Stanley cleared his throat and his next words stayed with Maggie ever after. They burned their way into her heart. Hope - was that it?

Stanley did not speak loudly but no one missed a word of what he had to say.

"Hear me, everyone in this room. Some day - and we don't know exactly which day - Maggie *will* have something to say. She will need her voice and she will use it when that time comes."

It was very uncharacteristic for Stanley to speak out like that, and the others couldn't help but see the tears welling up in his eyes. The silence that followed was awkward. Stanley added very softly, "Mark my words."

Always quick to share tears or laughter, Bessie's eyes were wet. She quickly got up and stood behind Stanley's chair. She gently tapped her palm up and down on the top of Stanley's shoulder. Through her emotion, she said very clearly, "Don't take it lightly, children, this kind of thing has happened before. When this man says 'mark my words', you need to mark them well."

Bobby stared straight ahead. His mood had been extra somber all summer, and this strange moment was unnatural. It felt like church. Hal's interest was piqued. He looked quizzically around the room. Maggie looked scared to death.

Hal was first to speak, his voice bright. "I'm sorry, Sis, I won't ever do that again. We'll just wait for the magic day Stanley promised us."

Bessie poured lemonade and passed around a plate of ginger-snaps. Hal took three and told her she was not only the most superior cook in the world, but also the most beautiful woman he'd ever seen. His remark broke the ice as he had intended, and suddenly Bessie's laugh bubbled up. "Oh, go on with you!"

Maggie later ran home for supper, but before she left she sneaked up on Stanley in the barn. She spoke scarcely above a whisper, "Tell me. Tell me what I'll say so I can practice."

"You'll just know, Maggie. There's no need to practice. You'll have some something to say. You'll know *what* to say and you'll know *when* to say it."

No one spoke of it again.

A TALK WITH BOBBY

Bessie rested her hand on her husband's arm as she poured his morning coffee.

"I had a talk with Bobby last night." Stanley was thrilled to hear that.

He raised his bushy eyebrows in surprise. "You did?"

"He came in late from the woodshop. It was hot out there and he came in for water."

"You were still up?" Stanley was eager for the details.

"No, but I was awake and I heard him in the kitchen." He poured us both a glass of water and we sat at the table. He seemed willing to chat. Right away, I mentioned him not eating."

He said, "Yeah, and that's kind of a waste since we've got the best cook in Saskatchewan right here!"

When I pressed further and asked if he is okay, he said, "I'm doing way better, Mom. Everything is going to be all right."

Stanley smiled, and Bessie continued.

"He wasn't pulling back like he has all summer. He was like the old Bobby. When I told him you heard the Higgins team are doing a sale this weekend, he said, "Let's go, Mom. You come, too! It's great entertainment."

I said it would be good for him to touch base with them again, and he agreed.

He said, "You know the auction is a world of its own. There's nothing like it."

Stanley was quiet and thoughtful. "I'm glad he opened up to you, Love. I can't seem to reach him, not after Cecil Grange went off on him the day we went for steeples."

"I think you'll find him different today, Stanley. He's at peace."

"Wonder if we should send him over to Fred's. He gets moody when he's alone, and Hal seems to be out of the picture now and stays in town. I think the boys had a falling out. Do you know anything about it?"

"He didn't say, but I doubt it. Hal's coming out today and they're working on name signs for their farm gate and ours. It's Hal's idea. He thinks they could make some samples, take orders, and make a buck on them."

"Probably could." Stanley gave Bessie a peck on the cheek as he turned to go outside.

"Stanley, here's another thing. Before he went back to his bed last night, Bobby said, 'How about a hug, Mom? It's been a while.' It took me back to that first day and all the days since…"

Stanley saw the start of tears in Bessie's eyes.

"He's a good one, all right." Stanley smiled as he headed out to the tractor. The hired man had set up a new ball of twine so the binder was ready to roll.

The boys measured and cut wood signs, tracing out the words, "Fiske" and "Andersen". When Bobby did two "Fiske" signs, Hal looked puzzled and Bobby explained, "For Fred, of course."

"Oh yeah, of course."

After an hour, the signs were taking shape. The letters were carefully painted and were set in the sun to dry. As they were discussing what sealant to use to make the signs weatherproof, Bobby looked at his friend, as if he had a sudden idea.

"Hal, I've collected a lot of valuable tools here. I'd like to give them to you."

Hal looked unimpressed. "Huh? Why? Are you retiring from the wood business?"

"I was just thinking, something might happen. I'm giving them to you, all of them!"

Hal stepped in front of Bobby and looked him in the eye.

"Knock it off, Bobby. You're scaring me. Nothing's going to happen. I don't want your tools."

The boys were satisfied with the look of the finished signs. Hal took the Andersen one with him to use as a sample for scaring up some orders. He had patched things up with the boss, the one he referred to as old Chrome-dome. It was true he also called him "Fathead", and the "Old Geezer", but Hal had managed to smooth talk his way back in and was slated to be at work in the morning. He watched the road to catch a ride to town with his mother's hired man.

When they heard Hal's ride approaching, Bobby was already walking towards the house. Hal called after him, "See ya'!" Maybe Bobby didn't hear him. He just kept on walking.

SOMETHING TO SAY!

The raised welts from her mother's hand were still visible on her cheek the morning after. Escape was on Maggie's mind as she quickly dressed and left the house. It was a balmy September Saturday, perfect for the harvest. There must have been frost the last few nights, as the leaves were turning color a little more each day. The maples all around the garden were yellow. The small chokecherry bushes had changed from green to fiery orange and red.

Maggie decided to take a day away from the yard. She wasn't sure what she would do or where she would go. No sense going to Fiske's, as Bessie was visiting the ladies in town. Her friend Lil, the one who arranged Fred's wedding supper, would pick her up at 2 o'clock. Hal and Dorie were at their jobs in town, and of course Stanley would be in the field with the hired man. Likely Bobby would be helping, too. That left only her mother. Not today!

She walked the full distance to the school, but she didn't go on the road. If someone saw her, they might see her face and think she did something really bad to deserve that smack. She found her way through the trees on cow paths she had never seen before. Never did she worry about getting lost, because she had horse sense. Stanley said so, because she could always find her way back, no matter what.

Maggie heard rustling in the dry grass near the path. She stopped and waited as seven sharp-tail grouse crossed the path in front of her. The brown and white young ones were almost adult size by now as they followed their mother in a straight line. They were not at all afraid of people, but continued on their merry way, even when they were close enough to see her. They looked like round little chickens, but Maggie liked them so much better than Thea's despicable hens in the chicken coop at home.

Some robins were flocking up, reminding Maggie that the summer was almost over. Thinking back, it hadn't been a very happy one, except for the day at the fair, and Fred and Colleen's wedding. She had written to her penpal, Pauline, a couple of times. When she first tried to write a letter, Bessie looked over her shoulder and said, "Land sakes alive, Child, didn't they teach you anything at school this year?"

It was hard to admit to Bessie that the teacher ignored her because she couldn't talk, so she simply let Bessie write both letters. She didn't even try to tell her what to say. Maggie realized she had not said a word, not even to Stanley or Bessie, since she trashed Bobby's cherished woodshop. She was still feeling guilty about that.

Change was in the wind. Hal told them he was done living at home, and Dorie had a chance to go to Winnipeg with her friend Jean. Jean's grandmother lived there, and the girls took the train, hoping to get a job in the big city.

It seemed all the woes of the world were on Maggie's shoulders that particular Saturday. It was an ordinary day, but twice she thought of the Big Clock. Every person she knew was marching to the tick-tock of the Big Clock's orders.

About two-thirty in the afternoon, she decided to head across the road. Stanley might come to the house at three for his drink and a snack. Suddenly, she was hungry, aware she had not eaten all day. She was well known for snooping, and had been straightened out many times for it by her exasperated sister.

"Don't sneak up on people! And don't snoop. Mind your own business!"

A light breeze rustled the leaves in Fiske's yard. The trees were dressed in gold and crimson. Maggie entered the yard and stood for a moment in the lane. Which way? She would never go in the house if no one was there, but there was no problem going to the barn. The Big Clock flashed into her mind and she blinked it away. She wouldn't go in through the big barn door, it was too heavy. She would just sneak in the back by the mangers. There was a little space there, where she had slipped through before to get inside.

She couldn't get over the quietness of the farmyard - not a bird, not a sound, just peace and silence. It was a blue sky day with puffy, still clouds. Without a bit of noise, she slid through the space behind the mangers.

What she saw froze her from head to toe. It was Bobby, and he had the gun, and it was pointing...

Her throat closed in. She couldn't swallow. Stanley's words echoed in her mind. "Someday - and we don't know which day - mark my words."

Maggie stretched her neck, and lifted her chin as high as she could to get some air. Still, he hadn't seen her or heard her.

"Don't!" she screamed, "Don't die!"

What was louder ? Her words or the deafening blast of the gun as it discharged on the barn floor where it landed on the wide boards!

Bobby was crying, down in the straw shaking and crying his heart out. Sobs tore at Maggie's throat. She threw herself beside him and hung on to his shirt. The heavy door opened and in came Stanley. Dear, good Stanley who must have instantly read the scene. He settled beside his son. All three were crying, sobbing into the silence of the afternoon.

Maggie staggered to her feet. She couldn't see Bobby's face because his hair was covering it. Stanley's arms were around his boy, so tight he would never let him go. Trembling, Maggie stared at them. She found her feet and leaned against the rough west wall of the stall.

I said, "Don't! Don't die!" She was amazed she could speak. She said it twice more.

Each time Stanley nodded, and new tears flowed down his weathered face. Softly, very softly, he repeated, "You said right. You said right."

Maggie did not remember much of the rest of the day. Bessie told her they were taking Bobby to the hospital "for his nerves". Maggie slept in her bed that night and spoke aloud into the darkness. Not caring if her mother was awake or not, she spoke clearly and with volume, "I had something to say!"

THE GIFT OF HOPE

There was a mighty stir among the members of the Fiske family in the days following Bobby's suicide attempt. His parents tenderly gathered around their son at the hospital, as did Fred and Colleen. Harvest was put on hold while they sorted out the calamity that had come upon them unawares.

Dr. Marshall, the now elderly physician, had fifteen years ago promised to support Bobby on his journey. The doctor had grown increasingly compassionate with the years of carrying his patients.

"Thank God!" he repeated over and over to his office walls, his head resting on his desk. He kept his patient sedated for a day and a night, and then when the boy was awake, Dr. Marshall pulled up a chair beside the hospital bed.

Bobby was weak. He would never forget the words that startled him and brought him to his senses. Those never-to-be-forgotten words kept going through his mind. "Don't die!"

"What was I thinking, Dr. Marshall? I wasn't thinking right!"

The doctor was gentle. "You're a sensitive lad, Bobby. We understood that early on. Sometimes we lose hope and we need help to restore it. The main thing is, you're safe and you're still here!"

Bobby had a burning question. "Will it happen again, Doc? I'm scared of that."

"Well Son, when such a thing happens, it is a real jolt and a wakeup call that never leaves us. It won't leave the rest of us either. You have an army of family and friends who won't let you go. If we keep things like this is a secret, it can take power over us. We will all be open about it, and we will be your support.

Bobby was grasping at every word. "I feel bad for Mom and Dad."

"No guilt, Bobby! By the grace of God, you are here, and that's all we care about. I need to see you every week for the next few months."

The boy looked exhausted, but he soaked up this reassurance like a dry sponge.

"I need all the help I can get."

"You're a strong young man, Bobby, and you need to be reassured of how important you are to all of us."

"Can you tell me why am I so tired?"

Dr. Marshall smiled sympathetically. "For two reasons, Bobby. You've had a severe emotional crisis, which is very draining. You've also been sedated to give you a rest after all that adrenaline rush."

Stanley stood at the foot of his son's hospital bed. The doctor reminded Stanley, "Let's not overlook the unsung hero who no doubt needs our help. The girl has suffered as well."

The next day Maggie sat in the big office, on a hard-backed chair where she had been seated once before. This time nurse Florence was nowhere in sight. Maggie felt small. Stanley had remained in the room at her request. Dr. Marshall removed his glasses and looked at her warmly.

"My dear, you saved a life. You will wear that badge of honor for the rest of your days." Maggie was surprised to see tears in his eyes. Do doctors cry?

He continued. "The Fiskes will never, ever forget what you did for them. You did a hard thing."

Maggie felt pressured to reply. She should say something - anything - to prove she could speak.

"I said, 'Don't die'."

The doctor nodded. "You did, and you will have so much more to say in the future. You have a lifetime of words ahead of you!"

Maggie felt scared. A lifetime of words to her sounded awful!

"You will have to force yourself to talk. That is the nature of elective mutism. The most wonderful thing is this, Maggie, you've now unlocked the door."

Stanley looked old and tired. He smiled at Maggie and said, "Something I learned a long time ago is this. When we help someone else, we almost always help ourselves. I think you helped yourself when you saved Bobby."

Dr. Marshall ended their meeting by telling Maggie if she ever had any questions for him, Stanley would bring her in. Maggie nodded. She would never come, but it was nice of him to offer.

Several days later, Bobby came into Andersen's yard, looking for Maggie. He found her planting some pansies in the corner of the garden. They had been growing in an old pail and she was giving them a better place to show off their bright yellow and purple blossoms. She dug a couple of holes and poured water into them.

Bobby spoke right away. "Maggie, you saved me." He closed his eyes. "It was so close."

She had not expected to see Bobby standing there in the garden, and she felt uneasy at first, well aware the last time she had seen him was the day in the barn.

"Come over to the house with me. Mom's making cookies." She dropped the hoe and they started walking on the path that led to Fiske's. What she said puzzled him. "The Big Clock didn't get you."

Bobby knew Maggie was an odd girl. It was strange now to hear her talking, as she had spoken only to his parents in her silent years. The first time he had heard her voice for a long, long time was that day in the barn, and now she was talking about a clock. He shrugged his shoulders and raised his eyebrows as he looked at her. He was asking for an explanation.

She opened her mouth to explain, and then closed it again. He wouldn't understand, and so instead she asked, "What kind of cookies is Bessie making?"

WHAT NEXT?

Stanley Fiske had a private talk with John and Ron Higgins. He sought their advice on Bobby's future. Should he go to Missouri for training? Or some other place? The Higgins brothers shared the options and their opinions. They had both attended the Missouri Auction School, which had started in 1905, and was the main training center for auctioneers. Both men said it had solidified their love for the business. After a short discussion they suggested, since Bobby was young, he could work with them for a year and then make a decision. In the meantime, they were well pleased to take him on as a partner, and they would pay him a good salary.

With that information, Stanley had a long talk with Bobby, asking what he wanted to pursue. Did he want to stay home and work on the farm? Did he want to work for Fred? What about Missouri, or the offer from the Higgins brothers? All the possibilities were on the table, and actually, all of them appealed to Bobby. It was like he had come back into the light from a dark place. He decided that for now, he would help with the harvest at home and at Fred's, and he would see Dr. Marshall once a week. No one was taking what had happened lightly. His emotions were at the surface, realizing how much support he had from his family.

It seemed strange that a couple of days ago he had *nothing to live for,* and now with a new perspective, he had *everything to live for.* The next months would be good, getting a fresh start and finding his way to a happy future.

THE NEW STUDENT

On the very first day of her last year at Aroma School, an unexpected event impacted fourteen year old Maggie. A fancy car pulled into the schoolyard at ten minutes to nine, and a tall blonde student got out. He carried a leather book bag and wore a plaid shirt and jeans. Though dressed like the other boys, there was something "rich" about him.

One of the Grade 1 boys ran up to him and said, "Boy, you sure have a shiny car!" The newcomer smiled down at the eager, little face and the others heard him say, "Oh it's not my car. I just get to ride in it."

Of course, everyone was agog with this unusual turn of events, filled with wondering and unasked questions as the school bell rang in the new term. Not very often did a new student show up, and especially when no one had heard of a new family moving into the area. The facts unfolded throughout the day. Victor Edwards was from the city and would attend Aroma school for the next school year. His father, an agricultural specialist, had a job at one of the nearby experimental farms. Victor said they were dealing aggressively with the problem of weeds in the fields. His dad's work would be important to the farmers in the whole province. He was not a braggart, they could tell that. He was friendly and looked like he would fit in well.

Laura and the other girls were already showing an interest. Maggie sat back to observe their flirtatious gestures, rather amused by how obvious they were. Maggie kept to herself and was considered a loner. After the noon lunch, she set to pulling weeds out of the dirt beside the steps. She wanted to see if any of the flowers the students planted in June had survived. Sure enough, when the taller weeds were removed, she found some blossoms. Violas (often called johnny-jump-ups) and snapdragons were struggling for light and moisture. The little area was looking better after only fifteen minutes of tending. As she stood to throw the pile of weeds over the fence, there was Victor, the new guy.

He disposed of the pile and said, "Those weeds sure take over, don't they!"

"They sure do. Same at home. I spend more time weeding in the garden than I do harvesting."

"You might get some help with that soon. My dad's work involves testing new herbicides to kill the weeds."

Maggie glanced over at the ball diamond where some of the students were playing ball. The teacher unearthed the old ball bag from the basement of the school. It held a couple of bats - a very small one for the little kids and a regular size for the rest. There was only one softball, a catcher's mitt, and a wire mask.

Maggie imagined everything must appear rather primitive to Victor, but he wasn't complaining. "Do you want to go play ball?" she asked, motioning to the game now in progress.

"Not really. I wanted to see what you are doing. Maybe checking out weeds runs in my family!"

She started in on the other side of the steps. The area she had already worked on looked really good. She wished there was water at the school for the suffering plants, but there was no well. A green army container held fresh water each day for drinking and for handwashing. One of the families was responsible for transporting it and was paid a few dollars a month for their trouble.

To Maggie's surprise, Victor hung around, wanting to know her name. They must teach them to be polite in the city schools.

Just then, they heard a girl's voice softly calling, "Hello, hello…" Maggie grinned. She knew exactly what was going on. Laura had put one of the little girls up to trying to distract Victor from talking to her. Oh well, no problem.

The bell rang soon after that. When they sat in their desks, the teacher commented on Maggie's work at the front of the school. Maggie's face flushed. She certainly hadn't done it to be noticed.

Plants called her name wherever she was - at Bessie's, or at home and now at school.

The new teacher, Miss Christine Clement, was a take-charge lady. "Maggie has given me an idea." She announced they should all come prepared the next day with garden tools and whatever else they thought could be used to spruce up the schoolyard. The whole area always looked drab and overgrown, especially after the summer with no one coming or going. Right on the spot, the teacher recited a poem by Rudyard Kipling, "The"Glory of the Garden". It fit perfectly into the discussion.

She added, "Tonight I'm going to think about what we can do, and you do the same. Bring some rakes from home, if you can."

A Grade 5 student raised her hand. "Summer's over, Miss Clement. I think it's too late to fix up the yard."

"Oh my goodness, Marjorie! If there's one thing you will learn this year and never forget, it is that it's never too late for anything! There's always time to try again and take another chance."

Her words hung in the air. They seemed to carry more meaning than pulling a few weeds around the dried out school yard. What she said about there always being time made Maggie think of the Big Clock.

At 3:30, the students were dismissed and rushed out the door, some to the barn to hitch up their buggy horses, and some to the gate to start the walk home. Right on time, the swanky, black car slowly approached the gate, and drove past the group of kids.

Victor made a point of running over to where Maggie was and asked with a big smile, "Wanna ride home?"

Almost before she knew what had happened, she was inside the vehicle, amazed at the plush seats and the fact that she was suddenly inside the car with Victor, instead of walking home in the hot sun.

"Gosh, they're going to be mad." She said it without thinking. He understood, and didn't ask who she meant was going to be mad.

"Don't worry about it, Maggie. Just tell us where to drop you off. Tomorrow I'll explain to them why I get a ride in the car. It's just that our new place is far from here. You know where the Experimental Farm is?"

Maggie nodded. She knew it was several miles away. "Couldn't you have gone to a closer school?"

"I could have. There are a few closer schools, but my mother knows Miss Clement and says she is the best in the west."

"So how did you like our school today? It sure must be different from the city".

"Well, it is different, but I like it already."

"I do too. I've been going for eight years, since Grade 1."

Victor smiled, "Do you have a best friend?"

"No, I never did. Do you?"

"Left them all behind. I wasn't keen on Dad's new job bringing us way out there, but there might be a lot for me to learn. I liked what Miss Clement said today, about trying something new and taking a chance."

For once in her life, Maggie was not stuck for words, and Victor was easy to confide in. She looked out at the fields where the barley beards were waving in the breeze. "Nothing new ever happens for me."

Victor had a lot of questions about how things were done in the west. "What about next year? What happens for you after Grade 8?"

"Well, there's no next year at school for me. I'm done in June. I'll finish Grade 8, and that's it."

A look of concern settled on Victor's face. "But, what will you do?"

"Stay home. There's always lots of work to do."

Victor still looked puzzled. "Don't your mom and dad care that you're quitting?"

Maggie decided to skip the details. "Not a fig. They don't care a fig."

The mile and a half flew by. She pointed to her driveway, thinking they would drop her off right there, but instead, the driver slowly turned into the lane and parked by the house.

"Wow!" Victor was in shock. The poplar trees lining the lane had grown tall and provided welcome shade. The yard was spectacular, as was the garden.

As soon as the car stopped, they got out and he took a look around. The dilapidated old house, with its weathered, brown shingles, was enhanced by tall hollyhocks in pink and purple blossoms, tied up near the steps. The door of the house was painted white, and in a rustic sort of way, it was a pretty scene. Maggie had painted uniform white stones to mark off flower beds. Sunflowers grew tall in the garden, turning their faces to follow the afternoon sun as it moved across the sky.

"I see your work in all of this," Victor said admiringly. He had been impressed with her quick work on the flower bed at the school.

"It's a hobby of mine. Work comes first, and then the flowers." Victor looked around again before he got in the front passenger seat.

"See you tomorrow."

Maggie forgot to say thanks, and she kicked herself for that the minute the car pulled out of the lane. It was so strange - a new, black car in their yard, and a handsome boy admiring her work. She saw her mother's face at the window. Thea would be wondering, too, and probably not pleased she had caught a ride home from school.

Perhaps she would have a friend her age at last. Could it be true? Was Victor someone who, for the biggest unexplainable mystery in the world, decided she was worth befriending? She did not feel his pity. There was none.

As it turned out, he was a friend to all the students and Miss Clement, his mother's friend. Victor was a remarkable young man who had the makings of a politician - popular, fair, and mature for his age. He seemed to have been raised with good values and he was respected for it at the school.

The students were allowed to eat their lunches outside if they chose. Most of the older students sat together in the shade of the maple trees that bordered the schoolyard. Victor was sitting next to Maggie when the trio of Grade 3 girls ran up to them and chanted:

"Victor and Maggie sitting in a tree. K-i-s-s-i-n-g!"

Victor burst out laughing, and said, "That's a funny one! Did you ever hear this?

The deer love the valley, The fox loves the hills,
The boys love the girls, And I guess they always will."

He effectively diffused the kissing rhyme and in so doing, won over the little girls in a heartbeat.

THE WORLD IS AT YOUR FEET

Miss Clement taught her heart out during her first term at Aroma School. It turned out to be the best year ever for Maggie. The lady had been teaching school for four years and was pretty much considered by most to be an "old maid schoolmarm". She was a confident teacher with a good mix of firmness and kindness. She did well with the little ones who were sent along with older brothers and sisters but should have hung on to their mothers' skirts for another year or two. Miss Clement also did exceptionally well with the older students, such as Maggie and Victor, giving all she had to infuse dreams for their futures.

She made learning fun. "There is such a lot to learn - so much to fill our heads with. Remember our brains can hold way more than we think!"

She offered endless possibilities. "Students, all of you never forget, the world is at your feet! You can do whatever you set your mind and heart to. This is a marvelous time in the world to be young. Everything lies ahead of you!"

A set of encyclopedias was placed at the front (not at the back) of the room and those volumes were her bible. Miss Clement's constant admonitions were, check it out, ask, explore, discover. Her theme was, if you don't know, find out.

It was a year of learning like no other. The younger grades absorbed knowledge as it fell on their heads from the higher grades. She covered poetry such as "The Yarn of the Nancy Bell" by W.S. Gilbert. They learned it and loved it and recited it on Friday afternoons, during the half-hour program at the end of each week. "Oh, I am a cook and a Captain bold, and the mate of the Nancy brig".

Miss Clement said she couldn't carry a tune in a bucket so there was no singing in music class. Instead, she opted for classic poems that fit the themes from history lessons. She talked of distant places far from Saskatchewan and the farm life they had known thus far. Victor, the new student from down east, was the exception, as he had experienced travel across the country and knew a little more of the bigger world.

The students studied in earnest. There was no time for the family feuds that had surfaced in past years at the school. Miss Clement held the key to learning as she created a thirst for knowledge, and the resulting curiosity pushed the children to seek out the answers.

She injected fun into the entire school year. The study of local trees was enriched by a school hike for all students. They walked a couple of miles in the area surrounding the school, making observations, and taking notes. She told them to bring their school lunches along and so the lesson turned into a hike and a picnic. The students made memories as they soaked up more and more of their lessons under her expert teaching.

Another fascinating topic Miss Clement taught was the system of land description in Saskatchewan. To her surprise, several of the students knew the land description of their farm off by heart. At her request they wrote them on the blackboard. Those who didn't know were asked to bring that information the following day. Maggie asked her mother that evening, but Thea was in a sour mood and said the teacher was poking her nose where she shouldn't. It was none of her business where they lived!

Maggie took a quick walk across the road before bed, and of course, Bessie was happy to write down the land description for her. So often the Fiskes filled in for what was lacking at home.

Miss Clement was a walking encyclopedia! She taught the intricate system of the enormous Dominion Land Survey, imagining with the students the miles of vast, uncharted prairie land. She gave credit to the survey teams who labored in beastly weather and treacherous terrain, ever pressing westward on foot or horseback.

The head of each twenty-man survey group was the party chief, who used with precision the necessary instruments to measure and map the prairie. The students learned the names of these items: solar compass, Gunter's Chain (for measuring), a theodolite, dumpy level, and an alidade. The teacher had promised at the beginning of the school year that the children would be amazed at what their brains could handle. Each day they tackled new information. The surveyors' work included marking road allowances, correction lines, and land designated for railroads, and schools.

One morning Miss Clement led the students outside to read the land description of Aroma School from the sign above the dormer window: *Aroma School District, 1920. SW 1/4, Section 11, Twp 50, RR 20, W 3rd.* The sign had been there all along since the school was built, but no one had taken notice of the numbers before, nor did anyone have a clue what they meant.

The students did not digest all of the information, but by the end of their diligent study of the DLS, their drawings were pinned to the walls, along with sketches of maps and grids of townships, and notes on meridians. They now realized that the mysterious iron pins that marked off their land, were buried like secret treasure. They knew the answers when Miss Clement asked, "How many quarters in a section?" or "How many sections in a township?" Finally, the students' farmland descriptions that were still displayed on the blackboard made some sense.

The teacher assigned projects according to each student's interests. Victor was given the topic of experimental farms in Saskatchewan. It would be his job to gather information from his father and other government staff who worked there, so he could later share his findings with the rest of the school. Maggie was tasked with reporting on gardens, flowers, trees, and shrubs. The topics were varied and suited to individual students. Some had an interest in cattle, the weather, and the royal family. Whatever they were drawn to, Miss Clement guided them in their work. Wolfie was only eight years old but he rode his little, black, Shetland pony to school each day, and the teacher helped him prepare a report on horses.

The youngest students were fascinated to hear about hens at the various experimental farms across Canada that were competing as to how many eggs were laid in a year. The children drew excellent pictures of hens and roosters and eggs, as they were familiar sights on their rounds of gathering eggs at home. It was always a race to find the eggs first, before a magpie swooped in for a tasty treat, unless the laying boxes were safely secured as they were on Thea's chicken farm. Maggie paid no attention to the topic of chickens. They were strictly her mother's domain, and the garden was hers.

AN UNEXPECTED JOB

Early in May, Victor told Maggie he had good news. That morning, he got out of the car and hurried straight to where Maggie was chatting with the littlest kids at school. Some time ago, Victor suggested she would be a fine teacher, because the younger students liked to spend time with her. She knew she was too shy to ever reach that pinnacle. A teacher needed to be good with words and had to talk all day long. Maggie was still not an "easy talker", even though she was relieved to have left her silent years behind. Teaching a school like Aroma that was packed with students would certainly not be in her future, as much as she would have liked it to be.

They walked towards the school together. "My driver wants to talk to you and your mother." Maggie's heart sank. Whatever this involved, it was not good news. Victor would see her mother up close and who knew what dreadful things she would have to say.

He explained the purpose of the intended visit. "The directors of the experimental farms are making deals with farmers in various parts of the province. They need to rent a portion of land for their small crop plots, and my driver will be making that offer to your mother." Maggie knew Thea would be interested in making a little extra money, and so she relaxed somewhat about how things would go.

Victor had a further surprise. "They have a job for you, if you'd like it." Maggie couldn't hide her interest, and he quickly explained. "They also need a person who lives near the crop plots, to record the daily temperature and the amount of rainfall. They want to hire you for that."

Maggie had recently heard about this. Stanley mentioned a couple of farmers who wished to be offered this opportunity.

"How did we get chosen?" she asked Victor.

He answered with a grin, "Well, possibly a little bird made a suggestion."

Maggie hoped against hope that Maw would be in a good enough mood to agree. Friday was egg day. Without fail, Thea delivered fresh eggs to the two stores in town. The familiar black car pulled into the yard and parked near the house, just as Thea was unhitching Old Nag from the buggy after her trip to town.

Thea wore a decent print dress with a clean, dark blue apron over it. To Maggie's relief, for a change, her mother looked as passable as any farm woman in the area.

The driver was a tall, dark man with a small mustache, and hair parted in the middle. He had never formally met Thea, even though he had been driving into the yard on weekdays for ten months. He introduced himself as John Roy and reached to shake hands. Thea mumbled her name. This was going well so far. Her mother listened to the proposal of renting out a small portion of her land near the road for easy access to the experimental farm workers and their miniature machinery. It would be called a sub-station. The idea immediately caught her interest.

Mr. Roy continued. "We have a further job which I would like to offer your daughter. At the Experimental Farm, we are always thinking ahead, and we know our young people are the future farmers of tomorrow. He then repeated the aspects of the job Victor had already explained to Maggie at school.

The tall man was friendly, yet businesslike. Thea didn't invite them into the house, or even to sit on the porch where the wooden chairs were lined up. It would have been a friendly gesture. Maggie knew other farm women would have started a fire already and put the kettle on to boil.

They continued to stand in the yard near the car. "So, Mrs. Andersen, do we have a deal?"

She jerked her head towards Maggie and asked, "Think she can handle it?"

"I have no doubt."

It was agreed he would bring the contract papers out the next morning for Thea to sign. The company had immediate plans to fence off the area for their small crop plots, prepare the soil, and get on with seeding.

Maggie was excited at the thought of having a job, no matter how small it was. Victor encouraged her that she was dependable and would be an excellent employee. Thea was in a fine mood that night. The prospect of additional income must have suited her fancy. Even though Maggie would not go to town school or ever become a teacher, she would give this opportunity her very best effort.

June came all too quickly, and as the last days of the school year came and went, Maggie felt loneliness building inside. Victor would go. He often mentioned now how he would always remember this year and how much he had learned. More often now he mentioned details about his city life back home. Maggie knew she would miss him. She would miss the other students, especially those her age. She would even miss Laura, who had come a long way in accepting Victor's preference for Maggie's company. The girls had become friends. Some of the others from Grade 8 planned to go to town school for Grade 9, as Maggie's sister Dorie had done. Maggie would also miss the teacher's kindness and encouragement. Miss Clement had met and surpassed her goal of inspiring the students to learn, and to pack in more knowledge than they ever dreamed possible.

The summer ahead stretched out like a long and lonely road. Maggie contemplated her future on the chicken farm with her abusive mother. The years ahead looked bleak and dark without school to brighten them.

The June days relentlessly ticked by, steadily and rapidly. Every day Maggie heard a voice from deep within. It was a silent plea.

"Stop the Big Clock, just wait a bit, don't let it be over." But there is no stopping the March of Time.

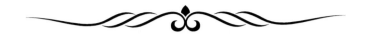

BOBBY, THE AUCTIONEER

Maggie often met up with Bobby during the first months after the day in the barn, since he stayed around home for the first year. He worked the harvest with his brother and his dad, then spent the winter working on his wood projects. He added a little wood heater to his woodshop and turned out flawless items for sale. Sometimes Hal came, and they worked together like old times. Bessie's friend, Lil, brought her grandsons over on Saturdays so Bobby could teach them what he knew about wood carving.

Every time Maggie saw him, she noticed Bobby smiled more and seemed to be happy with his life. During that first winter, he offered to play checkers with her when she visited at their house. He carved an exquisite horse as a Christmas gift to her. Bobby would always hold a soft spot in his heart for the girl who saved his life.

Springtime was the beginning of auction season, and the Higgins Brothers lost no time in making contact. Did he want to hire on for the season? They also mentioned there were indoor sales in fall and winter if he wanted to travel with them when summer was over. For now, they were eager to add him to their staff for the upcoming farm sales in the area.

They were taken with the particular pitch of his chant and the nasal edge to it that lent itself to a unique auctioneer voice. Bobby was easy to listen to. His voice had the semblance of a microphone and the sound carried well.

Bobby was also good with numbers and aware of the bidders. His deadpan facial expression contrasted with the excitement in his voice as he described each item, and kept up the steady rhythm, captivating his bidders.

John Higgins was a believer in keeping up the pace and could be seen rapidly cranking his hand in a circle when Bobby was in the auctioneer seat. The psychological aspect of the chant engaged the bidders, relaying that "now or never" bidding urgency! Bobby had a natural bent for sizing up the crowd. Whether selling cars or farm machinery, his rhythm and roll kept the bidders on their toes.

Sometimes the Higgins brothers let Hal sell a few items, to keep him on his toes, they said. It was true the crowd liked Hal as he told jokes and dazzled them with his good-looking grin. But it was Bobby who drew them in with his dark eyes and characteristic sound. His cowboy hat was low. He did not attempt to win people over with winks or gestures, which worked in his favor as his serious demeanor presented a sense of honesty. He was not a smooth talker, but gave the impression he was giving them a square deal.

"Ladies and gentlemen. Ten dollars and go. I'm bid at ten dollars now - I'm bid at fifteen now - I'm bid at twenty now." He kept track of the bids like a pro right from the start.

As Bobby's auctioneer career took off, he became more confident and outgoing. Could this be the same young man who had no hope when he was fifteen years old? His outlook had changed from night to day. What had made the difference? At last he grasped the fact he was no better and no worse than anyone else. He also finally got it through his head that he meant the world to his family and friends.

The Big Clock kept track of the Fiskes and the Andersens as the years passed. Seconds, minutes, days, weeks, months, and years - meticulously recorded - the good and the bad, the happy and the sad. Every detail was documented as the pendulum swung back and forth, tick-tock, tick-tock.

JUST ANOTHER HARVEST

His name was Clay. In the fall of 1952, he joined the long list of hired men who had worked for Thea Andersen, fall and spring, over the years. She figured Hal might come to his senses and return home from his big city life to lend a hand. But Hal had very few good memories of home. He was making his way as a used car salesman, doing a little auction work on the side. He planned to develop a business auctioning off the used cars, which would eliminate the control of a boss. Hal had never responded well to working under anyone. He wished to have his own business, as Bobby Fiske had now had, but time would tell. He believed in himself, but he did not believe in taking his mother's orders, ever.

Thea was pleased when a beat-up truck barreled into the yard in response to an ad she had placed in the paper. A young man with a rough beard sat behind the wheel with a wife and kid beside him. He introduced himself as Clayton Barns.

Thea sized him up. She was left to make the decision alone, as Maggie was at Fiske's helping Bessie with canning. It wasn't much of a decision, as harvest was upon them already, and she was desperate. Besides, she was well aware she likely had earned a poor reputation as an employer. A former hired man had quit in the middle of seeding after a vicious altercation with Thea over spilled purple gas. He left the yard, cursing out of the open window of his truck. His sentiments were matched by her own well-chosen words and the shaking of her fist.

So far, Clayton sounded like a good bet. He said he had read her ad and was a hard worker, and he promised to stay till harvest was over. They discussed wages and meals. She directed him to go take a look at the bunkhouse where he would be staying. It was a small shed out near the chicken barn, but it was clean and neat, with a made-up bed, a window with no screen, some hooks on the wall, a basin and washstand. That was about it.

The wife got out of the truck to accompany him on his mission. She was small of stature, with poor posture, shoulders bent forward and her back curved. She wore a kerchief that showed a fringe of straw-colored hair around the edges. She lugged the heavy child, who was almost as big as she was. Thea noticed the chunky boy was not wearing shoes, which may have been why his mother didn't make him walk. The path to the bunkhouse was strewn with small stones and thistles, but Clayton didn't offer to carry the kid.

When they returned, Thea was sitting on the step, waiting. With a ready smile, the prospective hired man said, "Well, I'm in!" They shook hands, and Thea told him he could start in the morning. When she asked where he lived, he said they were staying with her parents. He didn't introduce the wife or child. Although he didn't sound like a successful, progressive young man living with the in-laws, Thea needed the help and he looked like he was used to hard work. As he headed back to the truck, he tipped his dusty felt hat in Thea's direction and said, "Okay, tomorrow morning. I'll be here by 6."

When Maggie returned, Thea didn't bother to tell her she had solved the problem of harvest help. Only when Clayton knocked on the door at supper time, did Maggie realize why Thea had cooked extra food and set the table for three. He seemed to appreciate a good meal, said thanks, and asked them to call him Clay, not Clayton. Thea shrugged at this request. Who cared what they called him, as long as he got the work done? His name was nothing to her.

Maggie worked out in the garden that evening, and she saw Clay come by with a pail of water for the bunkhouse. He set down the pail, grinned, and asked her name. There had been no introductions at the table.

"Maggie," she said simply, and then turned back to the row of carrots she was pulling out for winter storage.

"Do you live here full time?" he asked.

"Of course, it's my home."

"Oh, I thought you likely had a job in town. You look like a town girl."

He seemed to mean it as a compliment. A town girl.

"No, you're wrong. I'm a farm girl. I have a job working for the Experimental Station. I phone in temperature and rainfall every day."

This was a big speech for Maggie. Her inclination to be talkative and friendly revealed her loneliness. It had been a long summer. Thea was in an ugly mood every day. Maggie later found out her mother was beset by gingivitis and had toothaches day and night. She often didn't eat at all. It was as if Maggie and her mother lived on different planets. Thea and her chickens. Maggie and her garden. Clay now was in the mix. He took his direction from Thea, but directed his attention to Maggie, especially in the evenings after supper. She took to being outside, and he took to spending a little time with her, chatting her up about this and that. He complimented her red hair.

No one had said that before. He shaved his whiskers and looked almost handsome. He said it was too hot in the field, so he felt a lot better after the shave. They talked about this and that, and nothing in particular. He didn't say much about his life or what he had done before hiring on. Maggie remembered the hired man, Riley, who had never shared his past. He then disappeared in the night, without a word, after a questionable visit from a man in a dark car the day before. She wondered if Clay was a decent person, but what did it matter? As long as he did what Thea bossed him to do. This was just another harvest.

It was the loneliest summer ever. Maggie had not heard from her penpal, Pauline for months. Bessie's diabetes had worsened, and she was tired and needed to rest in the afternoons. Maggie often helped prepare supper for Stanley and their hired man, but she always returned home to eat. Clay turned out to be quite entertaining. He knew a few jokes, and even got Thea laughing one evening when she was feeling better.

His evening visits in the yard lasted longer and his compliments were more lavish. Maggie felt silly when he told her she was pretty. She knew it wasn't true, but heck, he could say whatever he wanted to. He would be gone after harvest.

One evening, Clay asked her to go for a walk. As they walked out the lane and onto the road, she noticed Thea at the window, looking sour as ever. Clay had washed up and slicked his hair straight back, and he wasn't wearing his old felt hat. He looked younger, nicer.

"You get lonesome out here, sometimes?" It was none of his business, and she knew that.

"Sometimes," she said quietly.

"Are you glad I'm here?"

"I never thought much about it."

"I'd like you to think about it."

It was that hushed and special time of the evening, when cool, fresh air settles in after a hot day. Shadows lengthen. Clouds gather for a golden sunset over the harvest fields.

"Does she ever go away?" he asked, nodding his head towards the house.

"Fridays she takes her eggs to town with the horse and buggy."

"Maybe we could get together when she's gone." Maggie looked at him in surprise. His comment was not innocent. She knew what he was insinuating.

"I don't think so." She turned around on the road, and began to briskly walk back the way they had come. The next night, she made sure she wasn't outside after supper.

He winked at her during supper the next night. "What a flirt," was her first thought. Her second thought was, "Well, maybe he does like me." That would be a miracle!

A girl with low self-esteem is a tried and true target for a man with evil intentions. The harvest months continued. Clay was a hard worker, as promised. Thea often went to bed early with her tooth-aches and headaches and whatever else she had going on. As long as the chickens were taken care of and supper made, she opted out of the final hours of the day. Maggie cleaned up the kitchen each night. Sometimes Clay sat out on the porch, waiting for her to be done. Each evening when she finished, he encouraged her to sit down for a bit outside and chat.

He promised he would take her away from this place. He had some money coming in from his uncle, and he planned to buy a place.

"I just need a little time, and it will all work out."

Maggie doubted him at first, but he was a big talker and had some ideas about the future that made her head spin. Imagine walking out on Thea - just on the spot one day, saying, "Bye Maw", and hopping in Clay's truck, never to return! It was a tantalizing thought, a dream that crowded out both her common sense and feelings of dejection.

By the end of September, Maggie had put the garden to bed. The Farmer's Almanac predicted an early winter. All the potatoes were dug and stored in the cellar bin. The work demanded plenty of digging, and carrying, and lifting, but it was done. Carrots and turnips were covered with sand, in their respective bins. Onions hung in bunches on nails hammered into the beams near the ladder. Maggie canned no end of corn, beets, peas, and beans. The rows of jars on the shelves represented many a hot day with both the boiler and the canner filled with sealers, bubbling in hot water on the wood stove. So much effort was required to prepare the vegetables, put them in the jars, and process them for hours. She also canned rhubarb, along with fruit ordered from the Okanagan and delivered to town by train. The beets had especially grown well in the garden, and she made a few dozen quarts of beet pickles.

It had been years since Thea had pitched in with the canning or any garden or yard work. That was Maggie's domain, and even though her back ached, it was part pleasure, part work. She much preferred outside work to working in the house. Thea was content to nurse her pains and take care of the chickens, selling dozens and dozens of washed eggs to the two stores in town, every Friday, without fail.

Maggie's flowers were better every year. Bessie had encouraged her years ago to dig up daisies, daylilies, and small lilacs from their yard and plant them at her home. She said, "It's called a friendship garden, my dear, and when it's all in bloom, you'll think of me." Maggie reciprocated with lily of the valley and hollyhocks, which had

113

always grown profusely in their yard. She and Bessie were friends, and their gardens were friends, too.

The days of fall had flown by. On the last day of October, Clay came in for breakfast and suddenly announced his departure.

"Time for me to go," he said with a grin. Then turning to Thea, he said, "Wonder if I could collect my final two weeks' worth of wages? I think I got all the work done up for you."

He stood up and stepped away from the table. Sweet talker that he was, he added, "It's been a pleasure."

"I'll pay you when I sell the grain and get the cash," Thea said shortly, disgusted with him for not giving notice before walking out. She had planned on him doing some fencing to keep the neighbor's cows out of her pasture. They had discussed it, but now he was packing off and expected a paycheck then and there.

"All right then. I'll come for it later, Thea," he said pleasantly, "That will work for me."

"It will have to," she retorted, giving him the darkest look possible.

Clay glanced at Maggie and looked embarrassed. "So I'm off." He clamped the old felt hat on his head and nodded at them both. His beard had grown scruffy again.

"Till we meet again." His truck rattled out the lane, and the roar of the engine was deafening.

A DEAL IS A DEAL

B y December, Thea had reached the end of her endurance. The old dentist in town pulled out every last one of her teeth on a cold and stormy day. Maggie had arranged for Stanley to take her mother to the dentist's office. She went along to make sure Thea was all right. It was the first time Thea had been in Fiske's truck since years ago when she had insulted their son, Bobby. Patient as Job and forgiving as a saint, Stanley expressed his sympathy as he dropped them off and later returned to ferry them home.

Thea was in bed for three days. Her gums had been infected and it was a severe ordeal getting over it. False teeth were in the future, but at this time her mouth needed to heal. Maggie looked after the precious chickens in her stead and prepared a tray of soft food for her mother twice a day.

In a couple of weeks, Thea was up and going again. She was in a more level frame of mind, now that she was not in constant pain. That is, until she figured out Maggie's state of affairs.

One morning as she ate porridge alone at the table, she asked, almost pleasantly, "What's with all this puking in the mornings?" Maggie didn't answer. She often chose silence rather than to get into a biting discussion.

"You pregnant or what?"

"Well, as a matter of fact, yes, I am," Maggie answered rather smugly, though she truly did not feel smug. She seldom got one over on her mother and she knew Thea would go crazy with her admission.

Thea stood to her feet by the table, her eyes blazing. "That devil of a hired man?"

Maggie nodded slightly.

"You stupid, stupid, stupid fool! He's got a wife and kid!"

"No, he doesn't. He does not! And just so you know, he's coming back and taking me away from here."

"You are beyond ignorant. He *does* have a wife and kid. They came the day I hired him. You were here - you saw them."

Maggie's eyes opened wide. "No, I wasn't here, I was helping Bessie that day. I never saw him until he came to work.

"I've got a good mind to shoot him." Thea's eyes were wild. She was known to be an unstable woman.

"Maw, you don't even have a gun anymore!" The truth about Clay was washing over her like crashing waves of the ocean. She was almost unable to breathe.

"Oh don't you worry. I have a gun all right, and I know how to use it."

Maggie stared at her mother who was shaking with pent-up emotion. She was wearing only her holey, faded nightgown that was tattered around the sleeveless edges. "There's a lot you don't know about me, Missy."

The next morning, Maggie saw a .22 leaning up against the steps. She wondered if it was loaded. She had spent the night awake, facing the truth. Speaking those words, admitting her pregnancy to her mother had made the whole thing take on reality. She knew very well that a 20 year old woman should have known way better than to be duped by a no-good, lying cheater. Throughout the night, she had considered her options. Her only choice was to stay where she was, on the chicken farm with her mother.

After breakfast, Thea gave her a vile look, and Maggie could hear her cursing just loud enough to be heard. Thea was winding up. Maggie looked warily at the gun.

Ironically, on that very morning, with the gun in place by the steps of the house, they heard the loud noise of an approaching motor. Someone was coming in on the snow-covered lane. Guess who…

Heart pounding, Maggie ducked behind the curtain, but not Thea. Oh, for sure not Thea! She was on the tear. She pushed her big feet into the overshoes she kept at the door. They had four metal clasps, but she didn't bother to fasten any of them or to pull on a jacket. Out she went down the steps, her boots open and flapping, as Clay cranked open the truck window. Thea could see the little wife and the child on the seat as they had been the first time that truck came in the lane. Thea's tongue was darting in and out of her chapped lips.

Eyes blazing, she said, "What d'ya want?"

Clay spoke ever so pleasantly. "Well, we came…" He said we, the nerve of him! "We came for my pay. A deal is a deal."

"It wasn't in the deal what you did here." Clay's eyes opened wide. Thea guessed what he immediately guessed.

"You dirty devil of a snake. I wouldn't give you a nickel after what you did. That bit of money I owe you will be put to good use on baby diapers."

The full realization of the truth dawned on Clay's face. You could see it wash like ice water over his forehead and down. The wife spoke up, her voice high pitched, "What's she saying Clay? What's she saying? What about diapers?"

In seconds, Thea grabbed the .22 and her flabby arms raised it to shoulder level. Clay rammed the truck into gear and forged ahead in the snow, trying to make the loop as fast as possible. Thea shot at the truck as it sashayed out the lane. The crack of the bullet sent shivers up Maggie's back and neck. Thea tramped back into the house, spitting and cursing like never before. Maggie escaped up the stairs and remained there for the rest of the day. The incident marked the end of the story, the final chapter, of Clayton Barns and the Andersens.

However, it was in no way the end of the story for Maggie. Thea badgered her almost every day. "You can't keep the kid. You've got no money and no home of your own. You'll have to give it to someone who deserves it. Someone who can give it a home. That's what people do, you know, stupid people. They go get themselves knocked up and then they adopt the kid out."

"I want to keep it," Maggie said, quietly. "I'd be a good mom."

"Yeah? You think a good mom!" On the few pennies you get from your little rain and sun job with the hotshots at the Experimental

Farm! You've got nothing, Maggie, and I will fight you tooth and nail to get rid of the baby when it's born."

The weeks and months went by. The quietness came again and it was easier not to communicate. Maggie retreated as the animosity grew between the two women. It was a long, cold winter. Maggie thought back to the days of her childhood when her mother had the pleasure of abusing her with a switch, or a stick and regular slaps across the face. Thea used different weapons now - her sharp tongue, her belittling words, her dark and disdainful looks. Maggie was not sure, but was it a possibility that her mother might someday load up the .22 again?

Amid the dark memories of her childhood, Maggie also thought back to the reprieve provided by the love and acceptance of the Fiske family. They were the ones who taught her what a loving family should be like. She remembered those two long silent years, when she spoke only to Stanley and Bessie, and sparingly, at that. She remembered that Stanley came up with ways to make her laugh, like the time he made a magic mouse out of one of his large white handkerchiefs. He folded it this way and that, over and over, till finally he tied two corners that formed little mouse ears. He then put the mouse in his hand and managed to push it from behind so the mouse jumped out at her. She begged to take it home, even though it was one of his best handkerchiefs. The mouse stayed intact for months.

She also remembered the unforgettable day in their shared history when she yelled out the words, "Don't! Don't die!" and in so doing, had saved a life. It was her only redeeming claim to fame. What would the Fiskes think of her now?

One day in March, she went to the doctor in town. He confirmed her guess of the baby's birthdate, about the middle of July. She planted the garden in the spring, the same as always. Nothing had changed, but everything had changed. Life would not be the same again. People would not think of her the same. She was now "damaged goods". Single men her age would not be interested in the likes of her. Old ladies' tongues would wag and her mother would berate her for the rest of her life. Her disgrace was a daily fact of life, constant and unrelenting, throughout that spring of '53.

Pauline's letters were once again frequent, and full of wedding talk. She was engaged to Nick Suberlak. He was the best catch in Saskatchewan, according to Pauline's glowing description. She asked if Maggie would be her bridesmaid at her spring wedding. Maggie wrote back and explained why she had to decline the honor.

Maggie had met Pauline's Prince Charming at a community ballgame in the fall and was in shock when she was face to face with him. He did not resemble any vision of a prince… and charming? Not so much! When he told Pauline it was time for them to go, she paused a second to make a final plan with Maggie to keep in touch. Nick narrowed his eyes and gave his intended a dark look. "I said we're going, Pauline. NOW!"

Maggie knew a long road stretched in front of her. Clay was long gone out of her life. Good riddance, now that she knew about his wife and kid. She suspected the road ahead of Pauline may be long and rough as well. On that day at the ballgame, Pauline hurriedly trotted after him, towards the car. She was so intent on trying to catch up to him, she didn't even say goodbye.

Maggie and Pauline continued to correspond. It always had been therapeutic for Maggie to write out her feelings, and her friend was eager to reply. They had more to say on paper than the few times they met face to face. After Maggie confided to Pauline that she was pregnant, she did not receive the concern she had expected.

Dear Maggie,

I am very surprised at what you told me. I never thought it would come to this.

These things happen, I guess. I'm sure not risking that before Nick and I get hitched.

What are you going to do?

I'll keep writing to you anyway.

Yours truly,
Pauline

Maggie didn't know what to write back, but she did affirm Pauline's decision. She said very little about her pregnancy to anyone else until it was close to the end and her worries became impossible to bear alone. The baby was due in mid-July and she had hidden her condition from everyone. She very seldom ventured over to Fiske's for fear of them finding out, but finally, she blurted out the truth when it was no longer possible to conceal. She had a feeling they already knew, because Pauline likely told Colleen. That kind of news takes off like wildfire.

Bessie gave her a copy of *The Canadian Mother and Child*, and Stanley was slated to take her to the hospital when the time came. They promised to be by her side, her friends forever. They were the salt of the earth, loyal friends, the kind that last a lifetime.

STRONGER THAN PARTING

The nurse came in at exactly 9 a.m.

It was the little dark-haired one, the nice one. She was carrying the baby, wrapped in a blue, coarsely woven blanket.

"Here's the little man," she said cheerfully. "I got permission for you to have him for a while. They said five minutes. I'll try to stretch that out."

Maggie reached for him. Not having held a baby ever before, she was surprised how comfortable and familiar he felt in her arms, even though he was crying as the nurse brought him in. As the nurse turned to leave, she encouraged Maggie, "Talk to him, he knows your voice already. And hold him tight. He's not used to the world being so big, yet."

The door closed behind her. Maggie looked into his tiny face. He looked like he was about to burst into more crying, It was easier for her to be silent. To talk was always an effort, especially right now.

She remembered Stanley's advice. "Don't be stingy with your words, Maggie. Don't go quiet on us again, we need to hear you."

She couldn't help but smile at the red little face blinking up at her with unfocused eyes.

"Baby…" She willed the words to come. "Baby boy…"

He immediately quieted. Did he snuggle closer, or was it her imagination? She felt the solid weight of his body close to her heart. Maybe he could hear her heartbeat, as he had throughout the months of being her passenger.

In her mind's eye, she could see the relentless Big Clock of life, marking this day, ticking off these five precious minutes that would come but once. She cleared her throat. She *would* talk to him, just like the nurse said.

"You and me," she began, and swallowed hard, "you and me, we could have made it good. The Big Clock was against us. The timing was wrong."

The baby seemed to feel the comfort of her voice, and surprisingly, so did she. "I'm so sorry I can't keep you. You're going to make it good with someone else."

Her next words came strong, almost angry. "I pray to God they love you even a smidge as much as I do." Tears were streaming, but it didn't matter. The baby didn't know, and she didn't care. She saw this date, July 15, on the Big Clock. It was burning bright and golden, sparkling in sunshine. This boy was not a mistake. He was a jewel, a precious gem who would grace the planet with his presence, and fill a special place.

The five minutes had no doubt passed by now, and Maggie knew the little dark-haired nurse must have been dawdling on purpose. The boy closed his deep, dark eyes. He was at peace. The wild beating of her heart was gathering speed again. The nurse would come. This moment would be over, yet it would last forever, somewhere in time.

The door was opening, slowly, silently. The young girl, not much older than Maggie, had tears in her eyes as she came close to the two of them.

Could a heart break like this without a sound? Why wasn't there a crash that sent the staff running to investigate the catastrophe? Could it pass without a care, except her own? This wasn't right.

She sat in the bed gripping the bundle, hanging on for dear life. Suddenly, strong arms went around her and her baby, and held them both as one, for a minute or more. The clock ticked off those beautiful seconds...tick-tock, tick-tock. Maggie's chest heaved as she tried to control the sounds of a mother's anguish. She slowed her breathing. She dare not waste this moment. It was too beautiful that someone was with her, to share her pain.

"I'll tell you something," said the little nurse, speaking close to Maggie's ear. She was still holding them. "You will never, ever forget this baby. Love is stronger than parting. Remember that!"

Alone, Maggie covered her head with the bedsheet and she did not move. The face on the Big Clock was smiling. I win again.

There was no reason to speak after that. The silent patient avoided the mothers and their squalling babes. She spent her time sleeping and gazing out the window. She was not looking at the buildings or the hospital parking lot, or taking in the city hum. The scenes playing through her mind were past and future. There was no present.

Past…Clay. Her baby was nothing of his, the soft downy, reddish hair, not Clay.

Future… There would be no choice except to go through the motions of living, but everything had changed. Maggie knew she would go home in a few days, and that was hard to think about. She would be alone, unbearably alone. She would once again be skinny Maggie, with no figure to speak of. Her ordeal was over, but there was no reward, and no hope for the future.

The yard would soon be dressed in fall colors, and the garden, as always, tucked away for winter before the snow came. She wondered if the job with the Experimental Station would be offered to her again. Maybe, maybe not. It didn't matter one way or the other. And of course, there would always be Maw and her chickens. Maggie was trapped with no choices.

It was Bessie who came in a few days later. With her loving smile and gentle touch on Maggie's hand, she said, "Time to go home, Love."

Home. Home without the baby. It was the first time she had seen anyone she knew since the birth. Tears were flowing.

"He was beautiful, Bessie. I wish…"

"He *is* beautiful Maggie, not he *was*, he *is*, and he is bringing joy to someone right this minute."

Without further discussion or conversation, Maggie dressed in the clothes Bessie brought from her upstairs bedroom at home. The green, flowered dress was baggy on her now. It would not take long to resume her former figure. Bessie brought a hairbrush and a ribbon. As soon as Maggie was presentable, they signed a paper at the desk and went out. Side by side, just the two of them to Stanley and the waiting truck. They put Maggie in the middle, as they had when she was a kid.

Stanley's eyes were warm and welcoming. "Good girl, Maggie. You're getting through this rough spot, and we'll be right with you in the days ahead."

He was offering a spark of hope. Maggie had no comment. There was nothing to say.

"You're staying with us for a few days, Maggie."

At that, her heart lifted. The thought of returning to gloating Thea and her snide remarks had been heavy on her mind.

"I am?"

"Yes you are, we're going to pamper you for a while and then maybe you can work with Bessie for a bit."

"How long?"

"Oh, we thought a couple of weeks. Would that be all right?" Relief splashed over her like a bucket of refreshing water on a burning hot day.

Maggie nodded. Words were hard to come by.

Stanley observed her effort. "Keep talking, Girl. Don't go quiet on us again. We need to keep you close, and words will help."

And so it was, the next two weeks passed swiftly and sweetly in the home of her friends who loved her like a daughter. The house was fresh and cool. Bessie had a way of spreading peace like a clean-smelling perfume all around the place. After supper, the two of them went for walks on the road Maggie had always loved. It was a well-used trail from behind Fiske's barn to the far end of the pasture. The grass had grown high on the sides with a ridge of grass in the middle. The evenings were windless and restful. "Restoring," Bessie called it. Bush rabbits were plentiful and hopped across the road in front of them. Stanley was busy making hay. He had hired a helper so that his work was manageable since Bobby left home.

One evening, Bessie mentioned that Bobby planned to be married. At 27 years old, he had devoted his time up until now to his career. His training at the Missouri Auctioneer School helped launch his career. He had become as successful as the Higgins brothers predicted when they took him under their wing. His family and his friends, including Maggie, had cheered when he established his own business - the Colonel Bob Auction Company. The Fiskes celebrated with a community party.

"He's coming home tomorrow with the girl. I really want to like her, Maggie."

"You will like her! Of course, you will. You like everyone."

"Not always, but if I don't, I'll have to pretend."

Maggie wondered what Bessie thought of Colleen, Fred's wife. She did seem bossy and probably was unhappy about not having children, but Bessie always treated her like gold.

Maggie asked the obvious question. "So if they are coming tomorrow, would you like me to go home?"

Bessie, sincere as ever said, "Actually Maggie, I would not like you to go home, ever. But I guess it must happen sometime. Thea is hounding Stanley nearly every day."

Maggie nodded. She had known all along it couldn't last forever.

"I have some advice for you Maggie, and this is it. Stand up for yourself! Right now, you have a fresh start. You are a woman, and you are deserving of her respect. Stand up tall and straight, and know you do not have to take her dirt any longer. She is a bully and a fool."

Maggie laughed out loud. "Bessie Fiske, would you say that again? I never believed you would say such a thing."

"Well, neither did I, and no, I won't say it again. I can't believe I said it even once. I'm glad Stanley didn't hear me."

As they neared the house on their return from the walk, Stanley was sitting on the porch chair, patiently waiting for his tea.

"I can go tonight," Maggie offered.

"No, you can't! Not a minute sooner than you must."

The sentimental talk was done. Maggie had one last deep, dreamless sleep in the upstairs bedroom that had once been Bobby's. The shortcut path across the little field to the road was somewhat overgrown. No one had used it much in the past months. She carried her few things in a book bag Bessie gave her. It had belonged to one of her boys back in their school days so long ago.

Maggie went up the steps towards the white door. It needed repainting. Her mother met her on the top step.

"Finally decided to come home, did you?"

"I did. It is my home, after all."

"What did he look like?"

"None of your business." She pushed past her mother and hurried upstairs to her familiar room. Everything was as she had left it, the bed still messed from when she had been lying there in pain waiting for Stanley to come and take her to the hospital. That was a century ago, a lifetime, sort of.

Her plants on the windowsill were bone dry. She couldn't help herself. She watered them right then and there and removed the dead blossoms. The next morning, she inspected the flowerbeds. It looked like Thea had tidied up the garden, piled up some tall weeds, and collected the cans with no top or bottom that had protected the tomato plants. The house was neat and had a lonely feel. Glancing around the farmyard, she saw Thea at the well pumping water. She never seemed to mind carrying the heavy buckets of water to the chicken pen.

"Those infernal chickens," Maggie said aloud to herself. Bessie's habit had worn off on her.

Thea looked tired. To be honest, she looked beat, and Maggie, with all that had gone on for her in the past weeks, had forgotten that her mother had her teeth out. No doubt it had been an awful summer for her, too. Though they lived together, each was very much alone. There was no love lost between them, as the saying goes.

The book Bessie gave to Maggie when she was pregnant was a newer version of *The Canadian Mother and Child*, published in 1949. It was a 232 page public health manual and contained charming black and white photos, illustrating the care of babies. Upon returning home from the hospital, Maggie's arms were empty, and she was drawn to the book that was now of no practical use to her. She studied the fetching pictures of mothers with their babies, wondering about her baby's home. It outlined the development of a baby at two weeks, at one month, two months. She followed along day by day, imagining a growing baby boy discovering the world. On page 80, she read about the early care of the newborn baby. "Apply warm olive oil, or other prepared oil, to the baby's body, except about the cord." She wondered if his new mother had known enough to do that, and did she have a copy of this book? She prayed for them to be decent parents, for love and every great thing she could imagine, everything he needed that she couldn't provide. "Please God, let him have it all."

The book included a section under the title, "Crying", in which Dr. John Gibbons wrote, "To develop a strong personality, a child must learn to take the rough with the smooth." Maggie pondered "rough" and "smooth". There had been lots of "rough" for her as a child in this house, and oh, how she wished for "smooth" for her baby, wherever he was.

Each night, before Maggie blew out the lamp in her bedroom, she stood by the window, looking through the shadows at the garden and the barnyard. On the prairies, the days are long in summer, and the light lasts a long time. She knew Thea couldn't hear what was said upstairs, but she spoke very softly, just in case. Two words, every night. "Goodnight, Baby".

IT SEEMS FAIR TO US

The Big Clock ticked off the days of the baby's first year. There was mystery underlying Maggie's thoughts of him. She constantly wondered where he was - was he nearby or was he far away? Was he healthy? Had he started walking yet?

Dorie had married two years ago and lived in Winnipeg. Thea waited anxiously for her letters and the occasional long-distance phone call. She eagerly devoured Dorie's letters quickly, as they were not long. Sometimes she left them on the table where Maggie picked them up when her mother left the room. Dorie worked in the huge Eaton's store downtown. The ladies' fashion department was just right for her. She had always liked the idea of being stylish and up-to-date. Only once or twice did she mention her husband, Paul, who worked as a mechanic at a garage not far from where they lived. There was never any talk of children and no mention of coming for a visit. She signed her letters, "As Always, Dora". She was no longer "Dorie", the nickname she carried her whole life as a girl on the farm. So she was Dora now, and she signed "as always". Was she the same "as always"? She couldn't have stayed exactly the same. Maggie wondered what it would be like to see her again.

Maggie knew that she herself, had changed. Since the baby, a lot had changed. Mostly, she was down. Nothing seemed to fix or fill the empty space in her mind. There was a feeling of despondency that she tried to fend off, but she wasn't strong enough to win that battle.

Once a week she went to Fiske's and cleaned house for Bessie, whose health seemed to be failing. She was happy to help out. It was the only day of the week she looked forward to, and besides the satisfaction of making the dust fly and leaving the house shining and polished, she loved spending time in their home.

One afternoon as she mopped the linoleum floor in the living room, she glanced over at Bessie who was gently rocking back and forth in the wooden rocking chair. Bessie appeared to be deep in thought. She smiled at Maggie and said, "What did you name the little man?"

Maggie leaned the mop against a chair. It meant more than she thought it would, to have someone ask. She answered with one word. "Danny."

An approving smile immediately spread across Bessie's face. "What a fine choice, Maggie!"

Warmth rose in Maggie's soul. Someone cared. Of course, it was Bessie who cared. She was the one who said long ago, "I love every kid on earth!" Maggie picked up the mop, cheered immensely by Bessie's inquiry. No doubt, known by a different name, somewhere this baby was bringing joy to a family. He was more than just a fading memory in his birth mother's mind. He was a real baby, whose days and months were marked as surely as everyone else's existence on the planet.

The Big Clock was keeping track of all Thea Andersen's off-spring. Counting their days and years and how they were spent. Maggie's job with the Experimental Farm had continued. It provided a little pocket money and a small amount of responsibility, which meant she had a place in the world, small as it was.

Hal checked in with his former home even less often than Dorie. He felt no obligation to communicate with his mother, but often sent a note to the Fiskes. The story was that he worked at a used car lot in Alberta. No doubt, he was up to no good, but whatever he was doing he was likely enjoying it.

It was a surprising development when Thea got word that both Dorie and Hal were coming home for a quick visit at the end of July. She wondered aloud to Maggie why they were coming and what they wanted. Maggie was curious and eager for them to come. Hers was a lonely existence. The garden and the yard were in full bloom the day her brother drove into the yard. He jumped out and yelled to Maggie who was picking peas in the garden.

"Hi-de-ho, Sis! What's up?" Maggie straightened her back and waved, immediately heading toward the house. At that moment, she noticed Dorie, who was just then climbing out of the passenger's seat. Maggie ran partway to greet her and then, as she got close, all she could muster was a quiet "hello". Dorie was taller than her sister and was dressed in a fine, beige, two-piece suit. She wore nylon stockings and high heels. What an odd choice to wear to the farm! Maggie was suddenly aware of her faded cotton dress and she realized she hadn't put a thought into ordering something new that would look attractive for her siblings' visit. Her mother, too, looked shabby. She wore an old, blue skirt with the hem down on one side. What a sorry-looking pair of poor country folks they must appear to these city slickers! Hal wore cowboy boots, a clean pair of jeans, and a short-sleeved, red shirt. He looked slick and his smile was as dazzling as ever. Whatever he didn't feel, he could fake and fool the whole world.

The meeting was awkward. There had not been enough caring or emotion expressed among them in the early years. Now they were like strangers, pretending they knew each other. Maggie retrieved the pail from the garden, sat on one of the porch chairs, and shelled the tender, green peas for supper. Thea had put a chicken in the oven, and pies were cooling by the kitchen window. Like old times. They brought out chairs from inside the house to join Maggie on the porch.

Hal was the first to speak. "Well, let's get right to it! You probably are wondering why me and Dorie came home."

The wish that they had come simply for the love of being with family evaporated like smoke in the air. Maggie's chair was furthest away, and she felt detached as if she were not a real part of the coming discussion. Silent again, she was intent on shelling peas, as Hal forged ahead. His words surprised the two farm women.

"I got a letter from Slim Webber a couple of weeks ago. The good news is, he wants to buy this quarter of land!"

A sour look settled on Thea's face. "Why didn't he ask me?"

Maggie had observed Thea was more edgy than usual these days, quick to get angry, and at Hal's first sentence, her eyes were hot and blazing.

"Calm down, Maw. He just thought it was best if he checked in with me first, man to man."

There was an audible snort from Thea, who stared him down, as he continued. Hal wasn't one bit bothered.

"I thought about it a lot, Maw, and then I got Dorie in on it. We both agree it's an excellent deal for you. You won't have to hire a man spring and fall, or go to the bother of selling grain, and all that goes with running the farm."

Thea stood to her feet. "You're stark, ravin' crazy, Hal. You're still a fool! Haven't changed a bit."

Dorie spoke up in a smooth Eaton's saleslady voice, "Aw Maw, don't get riled up. It's a big load for you to run this place. You're not getting any younger and this could be your chance to sell. Think of it this way, how many other offers have you had?"

Thea snapped back, "None, of course, because this farm's not for sale!"

Maggie continued to stare at them, her hands resting on the edges of the bowl of peas. Even though Hal and Dorie's proposal hugely affected her personally, she was a spectator on the edge of the family, as she had always been.

Hal was turning on the charm that had once worked so well on his mother. It was as if he and his sister had planned their presentation.

"He's offering a pretty penny for the quarter section, Maw. It would be plenty for you to live on. I already arranged with him to divide off the farmyard so you could have the house."

"Well, ain't that nice of you!" Thea said sarcastically.

Dorie took up her part again. "Think about it, Maw. Hal and I are concerned for you, as to how you're getting on out here. I know how much it means to you to still have your chickens."

"And what about her?" Thea pointed with her thumb to the end of the porch. All three turned their attention to the empty chair, the bowl of peas and the spilled pail of pea pods. Maggie was no longer there.

Thea, already rattled by the pressure from her two oldest, muttered loud enough for them to hear, "She's run off again, like always." She added resentfully, "Still goes to Fiske's."

Dorie leaned back on the straight-backed chair and looked out towards the garden lined by maple trees. "She has nowhere else, Maw. She has nowhere else."

Only three sat at the table for supper in the Andersen kitchen. Maggie must have returned sometime after dark. By breakfast time, she had set the table, and coffee was brewing.

Dorie came into the room, stretching her long arms over her head. She was wearing a short, silk duster. "Aw, Maggie, you're a dear. You've made scrambled eggs and toast."

Maggie smiled. "I did. Goodness knows we've got enough eggs around here to feed half the country."

It was a meal that would not be consumed. Angry voices could be heard out in the yard, and as Hal and Thea neared the house the air was blue with nasty words from both of them. It reminded Maggie of the day Thea had sent Clay Barns packing, cursing him right out of the yard, with a bullet zinging over the truck cab for good measure.

Thea's tongue was shooting in and out of her mouth and her whole body was vibrating. "You ain't getting a cent, Hal. You always were too big for your britches."

Maggie raised her eyebrows at her sister. She still looked like Dorie, not the sophisticated city woman named Dora that she pretended to be.

In all her life, Dorie never hesitated to speak up. She explained, "Well, Hal and I figure Maw should take the money from selling the land, and split it three ways. Hal, me and you guys."

Maggie's eyes turned into slits as if trying to comprehend what had just been said. "But that cuts me out."

"Oh, come on! You get to stay here and live here. What more could you expect?" She raised her voice then. "It's like we're dividing it into three households."

High and mighty old Dorie, same as always. Yes, "as always", the way she signed her letters. She hadn't changed at all.

She added coldly, "It seems fair to us, Maggie."

The yelling and cursing continued as Hal and Thea approached the steps. Suddenly, Thea tore into the house and Maggie knew exactly where she was going. She had witnessed that look before.

"Quick, you guys, she's going for the gun!"

Hal's busy tongue stopped mid-sentence. The keys he had been jingling annoyingly in his pocket since he arrived, suddenly came out as he high-tailed it to the car. Dorie realized they could well be in danger. She flew off the steps in a cloud of pink silk and landed in the passenger seat of Hal's shiny car.

Sure enough, and without a minute to spare, the gun was pointed at the rear end of the car as Hal goosed the engine and fishtailed out the lane, dust flying. There was more than dust in the air. Thea's cursing was something to behold. She looked like a crazy woman brandishing the gun at the lane, after shooting it into the air.

"Put that gun away!" Maggie spoke clearly and sternly. "Settle down, Maw." Thea dropped the gun on the ground and landed heavily in the nearest chair on the porch.

She was panting. "And to think I raised those two devils!"

"Calm down, Maw. Breathe deep - I'll get you a coffee."

They sat there on the hard chairs, letting the silence absorb the electricity in the air. Thea closed her eyes and leaned her head back. Without looking at her daughter she said, "And I thought you were the worst of the bunch."

The altercation had left Maggie spent and in shock. "I never tried to be the worst, Maw."

"I know that now." Thea still hadn't opened her eyes.

Maggie took charge. "One thing for sure, we have to get rid of the gun. This is twice now, Maw. What if you kill somebody!"

Thea's chest was still heaving, her tongue darting in and out. "Do you know what they're up to? They want me to sell out and they get most of the money! Stinking rats!"

Maggie nodded. "I know, Dorie told me. She said it seems fair to them."

"They ain't getting it, Maggie, not a red cent. I'll leave it all to you!"

Maggie was loathe to touch a gun. She had vowed never to do so that day in the barn when the Big Clock almost struck Bobby Fiske's final second. Could she do it? Taking a deep breath she marched down the steps and hesitantly wrapped the fingers of both hands around the smooth wood.

Thea called from her place on the porch. "It's not gonna bite you, it ain't loaded. Not anymore!"

Maggie carried the loathsome thing, pointing straight down towards the ground as Bobby had taught her to carry a sharp knife when she was a little girl. It was a sight for Stanley Fiske taking his morning cup of coffee at the breakfast table. Through the window, he first saw a flashy car tear down the road past their house, followed by a familiar figure coming across the field and down the path. She was gingerly carrying a .22, aimed at the ground. Bessie was first out the door, with Stanley close behind. As Maggie approached, Stanley took the gun.

"Get that thing away from me," Maggie said, tears welling up.

Stanley took it from her. "Your Maw been shooting at that hawk again?"

Maggie grinned ruefully, "No, this time, she took a pot shot at a couple of skunks!"

RISK AND HOPE

The Andersen family was irreparably fractured, finally finished once and for all. No more letters came from Winnipeg. Lady Dora from Eaton's Department Store had paid her last visit to her humble beginnings. Hal also made himself scarce - back to Alberta, hawking cars.

For the next few weeks, Thea was a little nicer around home, and put some effort into conversation with Maggie about the garden, canning, and the upcoming sale of her chickens. Neither woman mentioned the issue of selling the land to Slim Webber. The topic was too volatile for discussion.

On July 15, the Big Clock had chimed once, a quiet and gentle sound, marking little Danny's first birthday. Maggie spent the day crying, off and on. Try as she would, she couldn't get past the tears. Her resentment welled up every time she looked at her mother. Thea was well aware of the date on the calendar and by early afternoon, she had reached the end of her short fuse.

"Buck up. Nothing can be done about it now."

"Don't you have a heart, Maw? Do you ever think what it's like for me?"

Thea drew her lips in a straight line. "What's done is done. I couldn't afford another mouth to feed."

There was no argument in Maggie. "He was so little, Maw. He wouldn't have eaten very much."

Months ticked by and winter came again. Loneliness set in alongside the cold weather. All of Thea's children had abhorred her beloved chickens, and she had preferred over the years to do all the work herself, so it was done right. It was plain to see in the extremely cold weather that Thea needed help to carry water and chicken feed.

Maggie detested the things and the stench of them, but she dutifully joined her mother on chore duty morning and night.

Dark thoughts of the future never left her mind. Back in the days at Aroma School, the year Miss Clement was the teacher, the students memorized grand poetry. Maggie had memorized Rudyard Kipling's poem "If", and a line of it had come back to haunt her.

"If you can dream, and not make dreams your master"

For years now, Maggie had been dreaming of escape. What if Aunt Marion in Stillwater showed up and asked Maggie to come to live with her? What if she heard, after all these years, from Victor who lived down east? Those imaginative dreams were exactly that - imagination, but they had kept her going. But since the baby, things had changed. There were no more dreams. She knew the signs were all there. She would become a disgusting, mean-tempered chicken woman like her mother. Could there be a worse fate?

By November, the yard was filled with snow. The famous Saskatchewan blizzard of '55 blew in on December 13th. Maggie and Thea were thankful for the vegetables stored in the cellar, along with canned chicken and fruit. It was a snug feeling during the unrelenting storm to know they could hold out for a long time, safe and warm, and well-fed. After three days, Stanley plowed out their road with his small farm tractor that had a V-plow attached to the front. His knock on the door surprised them. Maggie opened the door and welcomed him inside. Stanley had come to check on them, to see how they had weathered the storm. He accepted a cup of coffee and hung around longer than they would have expected.

Finally, he headed for the door and pulled on his warm boots. He reached into his front overall pocket and cleared his throat. "Colleen sent you a letter, Maggie." Maggie realized later, he had been waiting for an opportunity to slip it to her when Thea wasn't watching. As Stanley passed the envelope to Maggie, he added, "Colleen said it's private." Thea eyed the letter as Maggie nodded to Stanley and hurried upstairs to her bedroom even before he left.

She expected the letter to be from Pauline, who perhaps had been visiting her sister. Pauline's wedding had taken place in June as planned. Maggie wasn't invited and she wouldn't have gone if she had been. You don't go out in public when you're eight months pregnant and not married. Since then, Pauline's letters were all about her fine wedding gifts, her cozy home, and her dashing husband. Maggie read between the lines, along with a little information Bessie had heard from Colleen. What she read there was quite a different story. Pauline was lonely, and there was nothing at all fancy in her tiny house, situated in her in-laws' yard. Her Prince Charming husband, Nick, went to town on Saturday nights by himself. Maggie and Pauline still corresponded weekly, but she had never before received a letter from Fred Fiske's wife.

Spending these winter months with Thea had worn Maggie to a frazzle. The woman was cruel and unbearable, and Maggie decided if this was her future, she would settle for anything in its place. Maggie had been feeling for quite a while now, that something had to give. Something needed to happen to break the heavy clouds of loneliness and depression that surrounded her, day after day.

It was amid these thoughts that the letter arrived from Colleen. Maggie read it several times. She did not know if it was a solution to her misery or a life sentence. She tried to sleep, but in the middle of the night she was standing at the window, listening to the wind as more snow swirled around the edges of the old house. She lit the lamp and read the letter one more time.

Dear Maggie,

Pauline tells me you're depressed and your nerves are bad. I am sorry to hear that, and Fred is concerned, too. A couple of days ago, I got a bright idea and I think it might be the answer for you.

Our neighbor, Robert Cleaver, lives on the farm a mile down the road from our place. The trouble is, his wife died last June, and he has five kids to look after. He tried a few housekeepers but they didn't work out. He has another one now but he told us she's flighty and he doesn't think she will last there much longer. When I heard him say that, I up and asked him if he would be interested in a marriage of convenience. He said maybe.

So, I told him about you, and that you're looking for an escape. I told him your mother is a miserable sort and you need a change. I said you are a hard worker and that Fred and his parents recommend you.

When I mentioned your age, he said you likely won't be interested. I hope it doesn't hurt your feelings for me to say it, Maggie, but a girl in your position, who's already had a baby, doesn't have her pick of the crop. I told him I thought you would say yes.

You are wondering what he is like. Well, I don't know his exact age but he must be in his 40's. I looked after the youngest boy for a few months before the new housekeeper came. He's four now, and his name is Mac. The kids do well in school. The oldest is Roy. Next is Will and I think he is thirteen. Nicky is seven. He likes animals and birds. The girl is eleven, and her name is Dot.

Their dad expects a lot of them and they work hard. Robert is not over his wife dying and he doesn't say very much. I hear the kids fight a lot. It would help them to have a woman in the house. There is a lot of work to do every day at their place but I think the older kids are good at helping with the younger ones. Wash day would be the worst.

We would certainly like to have you for a neighbor. I get lonely here myself, as most of the farms are far apart. Fred says I have to learn to drive so I can get around on my own.

Please think things over about Cleavers, and let us know soon.

Your friend,
Colleen Fiske

PS I asked Robert what to tell you about the kids. He said to say that Dot loves to read.

Life went on as usual in the days following, although Maggie's thoughts were whirling in crazy circles. They were invited to join the Fiskes for turkey dinner on Christmas Day. Maggie knew her mother wouldn't go, so she refused their kind invitation and asked to come instead on Boxing Day.

On Christmas morning, while Thea was outside feeding her chickens, Maggie cranked out one long, and two shorts on the phone. Bessie answered with a hearty "Merry Christmas!" Maggie asked if Colleen and Fred had arrived.

The answer was, "Yes, they sure did, but they have to get home before dark. Do you wish to speak to Colleen?" Apparently, Bessie was in on the plan.

"I have a letter for her."

"They'll stop in for it, Maggie. That's the best way."

Later, Fred's truck roared into the yard. Thea was on her way back to the house after the end-of-the-day chicken chores. She looked like a stuffed scarecrow with layers of coats and a toque pulled down over her eyes. Maggie met Fred as he got out of the truck, and she gave him the letter containing her answer.

"Merry Christmas and Happy New Year, Maggie!" Fred called, as he kicked the snow off the running board and climbed back into the truck. He would always be Maggie's hero. He was a sort of big brother to her. Colleen waved through the truck window. Maggie could just see a bit of her face through the little hole where the frost had been scraped away. Maggie shivered her way back into the house just as Thea removed her boots and layers of outdoor clothes.

"More secret letters?" she sneered.

Maggie smiled like a Cheshire cat. It was the first control she'd had in her world since before she gave away her baby.

"Kind of looks that way, doesn't it!"

A MARRIAGE OF CONVENIENCE

As it turned out, things happened sooner than planned. Colleen wrote a second letter, pleased as punch that Maggie had said yes. The latest news was that Robert Cleaver was willing to wait till spring unless his current housekeeper quit before then. He suggested that would give him a chance to meet Maggie a time or two, and as he put it, see if she was willing to put up with an old guy like him. It was an unusual arrangement that had been proposed, but Colleen was thrilled to see the plan shaping up.

She repeated what she had said in the first letter, that Robert's five children were good kids, and knew how to work. She said Robert was quiet and didn't talk much. "So that makes two of you," Colleen wrote.

Right after that letter arrived, the phone rang. No more dallying around and waiting till spring! It was Colleen on the line with the urgent information that the housekeeper at Cleavers was no more. How about this Saturday? Was she willing to take the plunge?

Maggie's side of the conversation was cagey. It was very important to her that Thea did not know what was going on. That may be the only satisfaction to come out of the whole thing! Colleen seemed to understand, and once she got an affirmative answer, she hung up. The message Maggie understood was that she should be ready from noon onward, on Saturday.

Upstairs, Maggie inspected her meager wardrobe. Dorie had left her little brown suitcase under the bed. Maggie carefully packed it with whatever was worth taking. It was not much. Well, maybe the guy is rich! Colleen didn't mention that part.

On Saturday morning about 11 o'clock, Maggie went upstairs to get ready. She brushed her hair and tied it with a blue ribbon. The line came to her mind, "Married in blue, you'll always be true." The weather was freezing cold and it was not a day for a fluffy dress, even if she'd had one. This was a day to be sensible and practical. She looked around her room for the last time. She had taken over Dorie's larger bedroom a few years before. Maggie felt no attachment to the room or anything in it. It had been nothing more than a place to escape from Thea's miserable company.

Thea stared in disbelief as Maggie descended the stairs with her suitcase.

"Are you crazy? Where do you think you're going in this weather?"

"That's for me to know and you to find out," Maggie replied smugly.

"Fiskes don't want you!" Thea shouted.

"I'm not going to Fiskes. I'm getting married."

The women heard the sound of a vehicle in the yard, Maggie already had her overshoes and her coat on. The last words she heard from inside the house were, "Leaving me with all the work, after all I've done for her!"

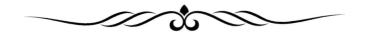

WEDDED BLISS

Robert Cleaver lifted Maggie's suitcase into the back of his truck. The bride and groom were both trying to get a look at each other, but there was not much to see through toques and scarves and heavy coats. Robert put the truck in gear and eased forward, laughing as he did so.

"This is the craziest thing I've ever done. How about you?"

Maggie grinned. "Same here!"

"Well, let's make the best of what we've got," Robert said, still with a boyish grin on his face.

Maggie couldn't tell, but she thought maybe he was handsome, or maybe he had been when he was younger. She was relieved that he didn't look that old.

The day was a blur. Considering the abominably cold weather and craziness of getting married sight unseen, reality didn't set in till the deed was done, and the truck was parked close to his house. He accompanied her inside and made a crude introduction to his flabbergasted children. "This is Maggie. We got married." That was all he said before he headed outside to the barn.

Maggie cleared off the table and one of the little boys helped her with the few dishes. Getting married to a stranger had seemed so bizarre all day and maybe even fun, but now she seriously wondered if she would be phoning Fred in a day or two and begging for a ride back to the chicken farm. She was between a rock and a hard place.

"The kids hate me," she said to herself, "and I don't blame them. They want their mom and I'm not her."

The rest of the winter was long. Maggie worked as hard as she knew how. She was useless at cooking but she was up to standard as a hard-working farm wife. The best times were when she and Robert and four-year-old Mac went to McKeen for groceries. She could pretend it was a date and could almost imagine they were a younger couple building a life together. But then the few hours in town were over, and it was back to the houseful of kids, and the piles of clothes on wash day. There were just so many of them living there. It felt like the house was going to burst at the seams.

It was better when spring came, and they could spread out into the great outdoors. Maggie had always preferred working outside. The garden, flowers, and yard work energized her. In the summer she rigged up a summer kitchen, where she could do the cooking and canning in the open space. Dot was a good help with planting the garden and processing vegetables and fruit.

Some days were good and some were not. There were moments when Maggie shook her head and wondered how she could have so completely taken leave of her senses on that freezing day in January when she walked out on Thea.

Maggie missed Stanley and Bessie. Finally, one summer day, she hitched up Queenie and took a buggy ride to see them.

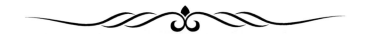

HEADING HOME

In mid-July, a horse and buggy rolled into Fiske's lane. Bessie peered out the window and squealed with joy. "It's Maggie!" she yelled, and then realized she was there alone, and no one could hear her. "Talking to myself again." She was smiling as she hurried into the yard.

"Let's get this girl some water." She was referring to the mare. Maggie and the buggy had a layer of dust on them. The roads were dry, and like the two farm women they were, they discussed the desperate need for rain. Bessie directed Maggie to park the buggy in a shady spot east of the house. Together, they walked to the well and filled a pail with cold water for Queenie. Maggie reached to carry the bucket.

She noticed the bruises up and down Bessie's arms. Tears came so easy now. Probably the pregnancy.

"What's going on Bessie?" Some of the bruises were old and yellow, some reddish blue. Maggie imagined all kinds of awful things. "Did you fall?"

"Oh no, it's those old diabetes needles. I'm taking more insulin than I did before. I'm doing okay."

The horse was eager to drink. She would, no doubt, patiently spend the afternoon in the cool shade of the poplar trees that edged the yard. Bessie admitted she was getting ready to go to town with a neighbor woman. They were invited to tea and Maggie insisted she not cancel.

"I have to go see Maw anyway, so I'll do that while you're gone."

"Be back here by three o'clock because you know Stanley will be in for his snack and a drink. You won't get away without him seeing you."

Maggie shook the dust off her light blue dress. It was loose except in the middle. As she freshened up at the sink and brushed her hair, she asked, "I guess you know I'm pregnant again?"

"Yes, Colleen told me. It's going to be better this time, I promise. Second babies are always easier, and this time you're not alone."

Then as an afterthought, the older woman asked.

"Is Cleaver good to you, Maggie?"

"Yeah, he is. I have no complaints about him."

"So what's the hardest part of living over there?"

"It's the kids, Bessie. I'm not doing well with kids. They don't like me and most days I don't like them either."

"Really? Fred speaks highly of them. He says they do well in school."

"It's not them, Bessie, there's nothing wrong with them. It's me!"

Bessie understood. "Probably your pregnancy makes it harder. Sometimes we get in a mood that is hard to break out of."

Bessie said Stanley and the hired man had taken lunch to the far field, so it was just the two of them in the house. Maggie made a sandwich for both of them as she felt at home in this house. This *was* home to her, in a way. The place across the road held no appeal, only memories of hard and lonely times.

It was not long until they heard the neighbor's car in the yard. Bessie had spruced up to go. She wore a print dress with pink tulips and green leaves, and before she went out the door, she removed her apron, hanging it on the hook in the porch.

"Do you want a ride over there?" Bessie asked, not wanting to walk out on her guest.

"Of course not. It's only a hop, skip, and a jump. I'm used to walking, and I think I know the way!"

Bessie grabbed her purse and got into the neighbor's car. She was still waving when they turned out the lane.

Maggie was in no hurry to see her mother. She felt like Goldilocks as she went into the second bedroom. A breeze was coming in the screened open window. The dark, wood dresser had a crocheted doily and lying across it was a fancy brush, comb, and hand mirror. It was a lovely dresser set with inlaid mother of pearl. Maggie immediately turned down the white, chenille bedspread with tufted pink and blue flowers on it, and stretched out on the blanket beneath it. She was always tired these days and it seemed a perfect opportunity to have a quiet lie down. There was no chance for that at home.

When Maggie awoke, it was 3 o'clock. Stanley was in the kitchen, opening the pantry door as he looked for a bit of something to eat.

He grinned when he saw Maggie come out of the guest bedroom.

"Well, hello stranger! I just asked the horse out there who had come to visit. She told me it was you."

The welcome in his eyes let Maggie know she was still loved in this house. He told her the binder had broken down in the field and the hired man was heading to town to get a piece fixed. "So looks like I got the rest of the day off!"

"Maybe it's your turn for an afternoon nap," Maggie suggested. Stanley looked weary.

"Oh no, I'd much rather talk with you. How's it going for you over there at McKeen?"

"It's fine, Stanley, better than there!" She pointed to her former home across the road. "For sure better than that."

After a minute, Maggie asked, "How's Maw?"

"Same as ever, we don't see her much. She spends her time with the chickens. She hatched out about 40 chicks this year."

"Really? She brought four broody hens over to me and so we hatched some, too."

Before she knew it, Maggie told Stanley about a recent incident that was heavy on her heart. What a big fool she had made of herself! It was the day Robert loaded the shotgun and destroyed the magpie nest out by the chicken coop.

"Well he had to," Stanley explained, "The magpies won't quit till they've killed every last chick and stolen every hen egg."

"I know all that, it was just my old fear of the gun. The blast nearly took out everyone's eardrums. I panicked and screamed at the little kids to stay in the house."

Stanley listened, visualizing the scene and understanding her fear.

"They thought I was crazy. I ran to the bedroom upstairs and shut the door, and then when it was over, I just couldn't bring myself to come out. Finally, Robert came and sat on the bed. He was mad at me at first and said I was scaring the kids. I almost couldn't say anything. I just tried so hard to get going, to utter even one word. Finally, I remembered what you said, that not talking is the worst, for others and for me. You told me even saying the wrong thing is better than going silent."

Stanley was an excellent listener. It was easy to confess her terrible actions that day. "Stanley, is it all right that I told him about Bobby and why I hate guns?"

"Oh, I'm glad you told him, Love. Now he'll understand. If we have the information, we can react better. Did you tell him it was the best thing you have ever done in your life? It took all you had when you saved our boy."

"I don't know if I explained it very well but he seemed to understand me better after. He made me come downstairs with him and the kids were all gawking at me, standing around. He gave it to them straight. 'Don't rile her,' he said, 'she's scared of guns.' I wanted them to know, but it made me feel like a little kid, for him to have to say that."

"I'm glad you explained it to him, Maggie. Good for you."

They were quiet for a while. Stanley was thinking over what she had said.

"Let me tell you how Bobby is doing now. His auctioneer business is making moolah, hand over fist!"

"Is he still nice? He didn't go back to being so mad, did he?"

"Honestly, Maggie, he's the nicest guy you'd ever care to meet! It took some time for him to come around. He just needed to understand that he's as good as the next guy."

Stanley added, "It's not the money, Maggie. I don't care if he's poor as a church mouse, as long as he is happy and doing okay."

"That's so good to hear," Maggie commented, thinking about Bobby's journey since the day in the barn.

Stanley smiled, "You've come a long ways yourself, Girl. We knew it was tough for you over there." He pointed in the direction of the Andersen's lane. "And even though we were sorry to see you go, it seemed like a better situation for you."

"I wish *I* were better, Stanley. They are wonderful little kids, and some of them are not so little. They're still so sad they lost their mom, and I'm a pretty poor substitute."

"You can't help that you're not her. Time is a healer…wait and see."

Maggie found her way along the overgrown path to her old home. She was concerned when she saw her mother sitting on the porch chair. It looked like she hadn't combed her hair for a week. Maggie hadn't seen her since the end of June, when she and Mac had returned the nesting boxes.

"How's it going, Maw?"

Thea didn't answer. Instead, she remarked, "Looks like you bin busy."

Maggie had no comment. Thea was referring to her pregnancy.

"I found a way to use up all those eggs you sent home with me last time."

Thea picked up her ears. "How's that?" If anything interested that woman, it was chickens and eggs.

"Ever hear of Denver sandwiches?"

"Nope."

"Well, it's easy. Robert and I had them at the little Chinese café in McKeen when we went into town for groceries. They're really tasty."

"You just fry up some onions and scramble some eggs, add a little cooked ham, salt, and pepper. I'll show you how." Maggie opened the screen door and went into the familiar kitchen. At least Thea was keeping the place tidy. Maggie put the kettle on for tea. She wondered if her mother was cooking meals for herself.

"Maw, you make some toast and I'll get the rest going."

In a few minutes, they were sitting across the table from one another, each with a Denver sandwich on a plate, and a pot of tea steeping on the embroidered tea cloth. Maggie had cut each sandwich corner to corner, creating four pieces. She stood two of the little sandwiches in the center, pointing upwards, and placed the other two flat on either side.

Thea took a bite. "Edible," was all she said.

"Oh, the kids love them!" Maggie said, "I make them all the time now." She knew she sounded like a real mother when she said it, and her conscience stabbed her. She wasn't a good mother. Making Denver sandwiches doesn't mean you're a good mother!

As they ate, Thea leaned towards her daughter. She carefully studied Maggie's face, to see how she would take the news.

"Remember that fancy pants kid that came to Aroma School that year? Well, he drove in here just yesterday. He was looking for you."

Maggie was in shock, "Who? Victor Edwards?"

Thea nodded, "I told him you don't live here anymore. He asked if you ever come to visit. I said never."

"That was a lie, I'm here right now."

"Well, you don't come much and you sure don't need him snooping around. Don't forget, you're a married woman."

It was clear Thea had never forgiven Maggie for leaving the farm and marrying Robert Cleaver. Maggie could imagine their meeting. Victor would be in his twenties now, the same as she was. She wondered what he thought when Thea met him in the yard in her holey clothes and disheveled hair.

"Don't worry, I sent him packing in a hurry."

"I'm sure you did. You're good at that, Maw."

"He had a fancy car, just like before when they drove him to school. He's getting bald. Fat, too."

Maggie tried to imagine Victor as a grown man.

"Why did he come? Did he say?"

"Of course. Said he wanted to talk to you."

"I scared him off. I told him you'd already had a kid and gave it up."

That stung. To think Thea would flip out that information as if it were a piece of news and a judgment against her.

Thea enjoyed letting out bits of Victor's visit.

"What did he say then?"

"He looked really mad and said, 'That doesn't bother me. I still want to see her'."

"So then I let him have it. I said, 'What kind of a nut are you? She's a married woman with five kids.' That's when he laughed like he didn't believe me."

"Did you explain?"

"Couldn't be bothered. I told him to move on. I said, 'I've sent more than one visitor off this farm to the tune of gunshot and I'll do the same with you'."

"Why are you so mean, Maw? Why?"

There was no answer to that question.

Maggie didn't bother to say goodbye. She quickly walked out the lane and back across the road. Dark clouds had gathered and she needed to head home in case it rained. As she looked at the sky, she once again saw the face of the Big Clock. Today it had the face of a gambler. You win some, you lose some. Timing is everything. Victor came too late. Way too late.

Stanley was puttering in the yard and welcomed her back. He realized she had to head for home. "Come on in and say goodbye to Bessie. She's back from town. Your visit has done us both good."

Maggie had more confessions to make. "I just need to tell you both again, I'm not doing well with the kids. Has Colleen said anything about it?"

"No, she hasn't. She wouldn't, even if it were true. Remember your new family doesn't know the rough road you've had. I do. Bessie and I do."

At that Maggie broke down. Stanley handed her a clean handkerchief from his overalls pocket. "It's okay to cry, Love. You're carrying a lot."

"I did the worst thing you can imagine! I told the girl I hated them all. How do I erase that?"

"Well, how about this. Sometime soon you say to that little girl, 'I'm sorry I said I hated you all. I don't hate you. I'm starting to like you more all the time'."

"Even if that's not true?"

"Yes, because the more often you say it, the more it becomes the truth. It seems to work that way. I call it the power of words. Try to make it right."

Stanley and Bessie waved them out of the yard as Queenie trotted briskly in the direction of home. Home is such a warm and comforting word. Home is where your heart is.

The evening was cool and Maggie suddenly had a headful of ideas, things she wanted to say to mend things with Dot. She thought about what she could say to the other kids. The main thing she had to do, and she resolved to follow through, was to open up and talk. Just like Stanley said, "Don't clam up. Force yourself to speak. There is power in words."

Bessie had filled a 2-quart sealer with grape Koolaid, and a Honey Bear pail filled with gingersnap cookies for the kids.

When Maggie came through the kitchen door, she was carrying the Koolaid and the cookies. She had been wondering all the way home what she could throw together for a late supper. The kids were always hungry.

Will quickly emptied the dustpan into the stove and set it beside the broom. He took the sealer from her and placed it on the table. The kids would like that. The house was tidy and Dot was finishing the dishes.

Surprised, Maggie exclaimed, "Supper is over? You did all the work!"

"Will helped. We made thin pancakes and strawberries from the garden." Maggie glanced at the chipped, green cupboard in the corner where leftovers were kept. Dot pointed to the stove.

"The boys ate about a hundred each, but I put some in the warming oven for you." A bowl of pancakes was covered with a clean cloth beside a dish of juicy, red berries.

Maggie was surprised at the extra big pile of rolled-up pancakes. "How many did you think I could eat?"

Dot grinned. "About ten - five for you and five for the baby."

STAY

If I could say just one
thing to anyone
struggling it would be
this. Stay. Stay the
course, the storm won't
last forever. I promise.
Stay because the world
won't be the same
without you. Stay
because even though
your heart may be
broken, you will break
So many more if you go.

Lindsay Dahlen ©2020

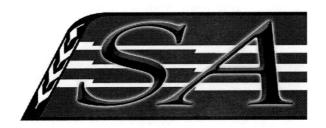

ACKNOWLEDGEMENTS

Thank you to my enthusiastic readers. Please keep in touch at dotontheprairie@gmail.com. and on the Dot on the Prairie Facebook page. I love to hear your feedback and suggestions.

Thank you to Lantern Hill Communications, for editing & proofreading.

Thank you to the "Thundering Herd" (as our mother called us) Trudy, Sharon, Jon, Le and Shelley, for applause and cheerleading, and for always being on my team.

Thank you to Sunny and Teddi, who created my practical, picture-perfect writing space.

Thank you to my niece Erin for support and assistance with the Dot on the Prairie Facebook page.

Thank you to my treasured friend Lindsay Dahlen, who has granted permission to share her award-winning poem, "Stay".

Thank you to my creative friend, Karla Nash, who dreams with me of future Dot on the Prairie plans.

Thank you to the artist duo, Noreen and Elya Foreman for the cover design on this book, Something to Say.

Thank you to Daylin Cooper, for hosting and producing the Launch Party

AROMA SCHOOL DISTRICT

1920

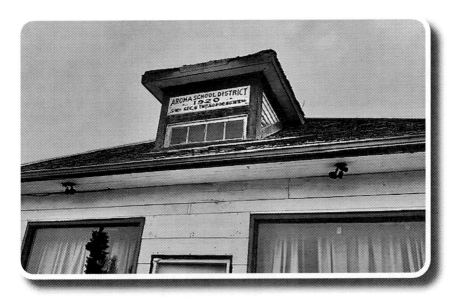

Land Description:
SW 1/4, Section 11, Twp 50, RR 20, W 3rd.

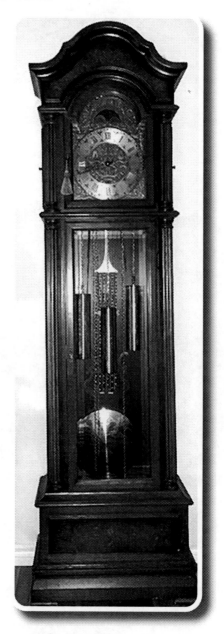

The Big Clock

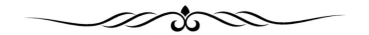

A NOTE TO MY READERS

The <u>Wandering Back to Saskatchewan</u> series has been a grand ride for me, and I am happy you are taking the trip with me!

I was asked recently about the process of writing a book. For me, the first step is to figure out the purpose. That's when I pull out my pen and notebook. What message do I want to convey? The story evolves later.

- My goal for <u>Dot on the Prairie</u> was to capture the details of life in Saskatchewan in the '50s, through the eyes of a child. I also hoped readers would find inspiration in the resilience of a young prairie girl named Dot.

- My hope with <u>Sure as the River</u> was to stir empathy and understanding regarding mental illness. My secondary aim was to carefully research and share information about hospitals for the mentally ill in Saskatchewan back in the 1940s – '50s.

- <u>Something to Say</u> speaks to the issue of suicide and depression, as well as the need to communicate and reach out for support.

- What's next? There well may be a fourth book in this series, but I am not certain yet of the title or the theme. Your suggestions and feedback are very helpful, so bring them on! Together, let's keep <u>Wandering Back to Saskatchewan</u>!